MW00647042

HASHIMOTO'S

Taming the Beast

HASHIMOTO'S
TAMING
THE BEAST

JANIE A. BOWTHORPE, M.ED.

Author of Stop the Thyroid Madness: A Patient
Revolution Against Decades of Inferior Treatment

Laughing Grape Publishing, LLC

This book is compiled to provide information only. Its publication and sale are not intended to replace the relationship with and guidance from your doctor, medical, or pharmaceutical professional, and it does not constitute the practice of medicine. The reader should regularly consult a physician in matters related to his/her health or symptoms that may require diagnosis or medical attention. You should also consult with your physician about any prescription drugs, vitamins, minerals, supplements, foods, or other treatments and therapies.

Neither the publisher, nor the author, nor any patient mentioned or quoted, nor any of the medical, health or wellness practitioners mentioned, takes responsibility for any consequences from any treatment, procedure, health modifications, actions, or application of any method by any person reading or following the information in this book.

Some names and identifying details have been changed to protect the privacy of individuals.

Every effort has been made to make this book as complete and accurate as possible. However, there may be mistakes, both typographical and in content. Therefore, this book should only be used as a guide, not as the ultimate source of information on Hashimoto's, thyroid, adrenal and related health issues. Furthermore, this book contains information that is current only up to the printing date.

Copyright @ 2019 by Janie A. Bowthorpe, M.Ed.
Laughing Grape Publishing, LLC
P.O. Box 2278
Dolores, Colorado 81323

Illustrations copyright © 2019 by Janie A. Bowthorpe
Cover and Interior Design © 2019 by Olivier Darbonville

All rights reserved. Printed in the United States of America. No part of this book may be used or reproduced in any manner whatsoever, electronic or mechanical, including photocopying, recording or by any information storage or retrieval system, without written permission from the author except in the case of brief quotations embodied in critical articles and reviews.

Library of Congress Cataloging-in Publication Data
Bowthorpe, Janie A
Hashimoto's: Taming the Beast/Janie A. Bowthorpe. M.Ed./Includes bibliographical references and index
ISBN 978-0-9856154-4-4
1. Hypothyroidism - Popular Works I. Title

LCCN: 2019903241 LOC Classification: RC648-665   Dewey: 616.4/44

Dedicated to

my Maine Coon sibling cats,
Jamie and Claire,

who while I spent a gargantuan
amount of time in research, reading,
evaluating, compiling and writing this
book, purred as they sat behind me in
the chair, purred as they laid next to
me on the couch, purred as they stood
under my desk, purred in the window of
my office.

Preface and Acknowledgements

As someone who suffered miserably for two long decades as a thyroid patient, then to see my life make a strong turn-around thanks to a better treatment with natural desiccated thyroid (which I was forced to find out about on my own) plus tweaking other issues, I was angry. I was angry that I went so years with doctors who knew nothing worthy about treating me correctly, and who were constantly telling me I was "normal".

So, I started a movement--**a patient-to-patient movement called Stop the Thyroid Madness, LLC** as expressed on the website, in the books, and on social media by the same name. And oh, how we've all come a long way with our combined experiences and wisdom as patients! We figured out how to get well!

And I knew, from all I've observed and compiled, is that it was time to contribute this book specifically about **autoimmune Hashimoto's disease**---an attack on the thyroid by the very immune system that should be protecting you. Hashimoto's patients have it rough—all the intricacies of an autoimmune disease on top of finding oneself with a damaged thyroid and hypothyroidism!

• *Thanks first and foremost go to YOU, the courageous Hashimoto's patient!* You have done a wonderful job over the recent years in expressing your challenges as well as your experiences and successes, so that others can learn from YOU!

• *Thanks to all those individuals who have websites about diet protocols to lower that autoimmune inflammation.* Some even have great recipes! There are so many.

• *Thanks to autoimmune-focused advocates who keep the information going on their websites and social media pages.* High five to YOU.

• *Thanks, in the name of truly helping patients, to those groups and their owners who focus on solid and time-tested patient-to-patient information from Stop the Thyroid Madness, like Jamie Dolan, the owner of the Facebook group called Adrenal Fatigue and Thyroid Care, or to the mods who help run the Yahoo Natural Thyroid Hormones group.* Your willingness to use patient experiences truly helps others.

• *Thanks to those doctors who DO listen to their patients.* Patients hope to see more just like you, as too many medical professionals are behind about putting Hashimoto's into remission.

• *Thanks to my dear husband* who always has such patience when I'm working longgggg hours, days and weeks on any book, and he ends up having to cook. He's diabetic and has done a SMASHING job eating much lower carb.

Janie A Bowthorpe M Ed

Table of Contents

a

Introduction

Hashimoto's (Hashi's) is an autoimmune disease. The latter means your immune system has gone beyond attacking bacteria and viruses—it's also attacking your own tissues and organs! *Boooo. Hiss.*

And it's a bit remarkable to discover that though there were medical suspicions of a body turning against itself for years, it wasn't until the 1950s and 1960s that the medical community was finally giving official mainstream recognition to **"autoimmune diseases"**, of which Hashimoto's is one.

In fact, this recognition now covers more than 100 autoimmune diseases—a number quoted by AARD, aka the American Autoimmune Related Diseases Association. And within this number, we know that most are attacking one organ in the body; others are about attacks spread throughout the body like lupus or rheumatoid arthritis.

The way to see 'autoimmunity' is that your immune system loses the knowledge that "you" are supposed to be different from an insidious "other". Of course, any harmful "other" with nothing but bad intentions should be attacked and neutralized, don't you agree? But for "you" to be attacked, too?? *That is an immune system gone loopy.*

And worse, the attack against "you" may go on and on before you even know it's going on! Those antibodies...which are supposed to be our soldier heroes, may be slowly building a "nutty" army against YOU without any symptoms...until there are symptoms!

So, you go about your life, either not noticing or misunderstanding what you may be noticing.

◆

And that is Hashimoto's disease.

Hashi's is about a psyched out immune system which begins to attack your healthy thyroid tissue, getting bolder and meaner about it over time. The attack is either towards the thyroid protein called **thyroglobulin**, which is the precursor of thyroid hormones, or the thyroid enzyme **peroxidase**, which also plays a role in the production of thyroid hormones. Or both.

And with that initial attack by a growing anti-thyroid army, comes numerous challenges by those with Hashimoto's disease.

Challenges faced by Hashi's Patients

- strange new and growing symptoms like easy fatigue and the need to nap
- the curiosity and frustration as to why there are more hairs in the shower drain
- the frustration of one's weight scale number going up
- increasing pesky symptoms like sleep problems, depression, brain fog and more
- the seesaw between feeling sluggish at times, then feeling hyper the next…back and forth
- doctors who proclaim you just need to exercise more and eat less
- doctors who say you need a therapist or psychiatrist
- doctors who simply throw an antidepressant your way
- a doctor who only gives you a hypothyroid diagnosis
- going to more doctors before you get the Hashi's diagnosis
- doctors who tell you to *wait it out*
- doctors who tell you *there's nothing to be done*

- trying to figure out how to lower those annoying overreactive antibodies
- chronic inflammation that only promotes more inflammation
- deciding which anti-inflammatory supplements might help or can be tolerated
- how to avoid flares from stress
- problem-causing foods
- the learning curve of eating differently
- how to get the right foods if eating out
- chronic and numerous gut problems that you have to learn about and treat
- how to get through any infection without feeling worse
- whether your Hashimoto's will pair with another autoimmune nuttiness
- people who don't get your problems
- not being able to live your life fully
- feeling judged
- feeling lonely and misunderstood

Also comes the challenge of working with doctors who have poor knowledge about treating the hypothyroidism you may now have.

What do you identify with below?

- being put on a poor medication like Synthroid or Levothyroxine (the body is not meant to live for T4 alone and will backfire, sooner or later)
- not realizing that though you may feel fine on T4, it's only a matter of time it will backfire
- being held hostage to the pituitary hormone TSH, which is the worst way to diagnose or treat

- seeing nutrients fall like iron, B12, vitamin D and more due to continued hypothyroidism which is lowering one's stomach acid— one cause of lowered nutrients
- being told by a doctor that your acid reflux is about too much stomach acid (it's usually about too low acid)
- doctors who don't test the RT3 (reverse T3), the inactive hormone which can go too high
- not understanding where the RT3 should fall (bottom 2-3 numbers in the range)
- finally finding a doctor to put you on natural desiccated thyroid (NDT) or T4/T3, but being underdosed due to their fear of NDT or T3, or worshipping the TSH instead of the free T3 and free T4
- a doctor who doesn't understand "optimal" in lab work (it's not about falling anywhere in those ridiculous "normal" ranges)
- acquiring a cortisol problem due to a poor treatment; being held hostage to the normal range
- not understanding how blood cortisol testing is inadequate (measures mostly unusable cortisol) and the need to do 24-hour cortisol saliva testing instead (measures unbound and useable)

More information in the updated revision book *Stop the Thyroid Madness: A Patient Revolution Against Decades of Inferior Treatment*

Having Hashimoto's is a beastly mess. But on the other side of the coin....

There is now rich information to help you reverse the autoimmune march towards destruction, to begin countering the inflammation, to identify, treat and reverse triggering problems, and to better treat the hypothyroidism. And this book represents all that information, plus references on where to go for even more information, aka Stop the Thyroid Madness website and books.

How to use this book

Get that highlighter! Underline. Mark the pages. Use every inch of this book as a reference for YOU. I have also supplied a blank page called NOTES after each chapter for you to write down important pages or to jot down applicable information in that chapter which applies to you.

Footnotes and Notes

I have tried to be generous with references/footnotes, showing you research, medical related articles, or good website pages to support the topic. Check them out when you want to learn more. If for some reason a URL changes over time, you can do your own internet search of the topic.

A focus on concise, yet key information

In this book, you won't see unneeded drawn-out information or stories. The attempt was to present that fundamental information with less pages to counter patient brain fog or problems with concentration.

The battle cry is this: *Hashimoto's, we are going to bring you down to your knobby autoimmune knees!*

Janie A Bowthorpe M Ed

Chapter 1

Immune System 101: When it's Good, When it's Not

Did you know that every day, there are all sorts of bad guys (antigens) in the environment) that want to get in your body and wreak havoc?

They can be in your food, on restaurant door handles, on gas pumps, in the air you breathe, in your kitchen sink. Everywhere.

If they get in, these bad guys want to move around in your body, hide in places, eat what they can, and make many, many copies of their bad selves in their path of destruction of your body. Sounds pretty disgusting, don't you think?

The names of those conniving bad guys are:

- **Bacteria** (single cell infection organisms with speedy little tails which can make you sick)
- **Fungi** (certain toxic versions of yeast and mold)
- **Parasites** (organism that feeds on you)
- **Viruses** (tiny toxic agents that infect/reproduce via host cells)

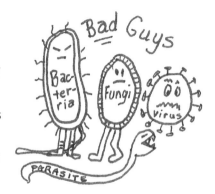

But voila...to the rescue comes a brilliant immune system.

First comes what you were born with as an immune system: skin to keep germs out, mucus to get them stuck, and little cells to overwhelm and absorb the nasty ones who get in. That mucus is everywhere, by the way—in your nose, sinuses, and even in your lungs. It also lines your stomach and intestines, and all the way down to the urethra and bladder!

But if that isn't enough, next comes a bad ass, well-oiled team of different white blood cells, plus proteins called antibodies. Together, they all do the following:

patrol
    guard
        recognize
            signal
                interact
                    activate
                        stimulate
                          trap
                            duplicate
                                call for backup
                                  devour
                                    inflame
                                      remember
                                        destroy!

The antibodies, which are like fierce little soldiers, are produced and released by white blood cells called B-cells. Antibodies will then multiply into the millions and bind to the surfaces of the intruders. Since an antibody is shaped like a little Y, picture all these Y's attached to a bad guy. That binding tells other cells to *destroy!*

There are different kinds of antibodies with different jobs, and that's where you get the names IgA, IgD, IgE, IgG, and IgM.

Geek Info About those Y-shaped Antibodies

There are five different kinds of antibodies released by the immune system, and they have different functions. The "I" stands for Immunoglobulin, another word for those protein antibodies. IgG and IgM can especially be exaggerated in autoimmune disease responses, and IgG especially high in Hashimoto's.

The five antibodies are:

- **IgA:** These are the antibodies in mucus membranes i.e. that which lines the interior of glands like the stomach or intestines, or that which covers the surface of other organs. IgA antibodies can also be found in your tears, sweat, or your saliva. These antibodies are always working to "neutralize" bad guys like viruses or bacteria.

- **IgD:** These antibodies are found in very small amounts in your blood. It has the function of signaling B cells, a type of white blood cells, to be activated, and IgD also works with IgM.

- **IgE:** These antibodies are produced by your immune system in a strong reaction to any "allergen". Allergens can be pollen, dust, insect stings, latex, different foods, mold and even pet hairs. These antibodies will travel to cells that release chemicals, thus causing your allergic reactions. Some examples of allergic reactions are rashes or hives, sneezing, a runny nose, congested nose, eyes that water or itch, or coughing. Or reactions can be trouble breathing, feeling dizzy, raspy voice, diarrhea, abdominal pain, or swelling.

- **IgG:** These are the most common of antibodies, as well as being the smallest. They circulate in your blood and any fluid outside of your cells like military sentries, watching, observing and ready to protect you by grabbing ahold of the bad guys. When they bind to bad guys, other immune cells are then activated to overpower the bad guys and destroy them. *These can be remarkably high with Hashimoto's disease.*

- **IgM:** These are the largest of antibodies and are found in all your bodily fluids. IgM is the first antibody to appear when the immune system is acting against a bad guy, thus making IgM very important in the diagnosis of infectious diseases. So, when they are found in your blood, your doctor knows they represent a *recent infection*. IgM antibodies act similarly to IgG antibodies in protecting you.

Whoops!! How your immune system goes totally overboard

Contrary to how elegantly and brilliantly a healthy immune system works, there is another ugly side of the coin: an immune system gone rogue. It's called autoimmunity--where one's immune system decides to touch the curl of its moustache and also attack your healthy tissue.

'Auto' in autoimmunity means "self", so the befuddled immune system starts attacking you, the self. It's an "abnormal" attack against "normal" parts of your body, i.e. your immune system is in a pickle...not understanding the difference between "you" and a "vile enemy"!! So "you", your tissues, become the target to destroy!

Most experts are going to say that they aren't yet totally sure why an immune system gets so seriously confused in certain individuals. But they do agree on the following:

- Genetics play a strong underlying role.
- Environmental triggers make it all worse.
- Gluten is especially triggering.
- Autoimmunity tends to run in families.
- Autoimmune disease usually pairs with other autoimmune diseases.
- More women than men have autoimmunity.
- There are at least 100 types of autoimmune diseases.
- Inflammation is a classic sign.
- Treatment depends on the disease

In this book, we're going to look at a particular autoimmune condition called Hashimoto's disease, the autoimmune attack of the thyroid.

NOTES

Chapter 2

The 10-Point Low Down About **Autoimmune Hashimoto's disease**

To be on the same page as to the subject of this informative book, let's first go over ten key points as to what Hashimoto's disease is about. You will also see Hashimoto's termed as Hashi's or Hashimoto's Thyroiditis.

1. **Hashimoto's disease is an autoimmune disorder,** meaning that while certain white blood cells from your immune system are producing protective antibodies to attack viruses, bacteria or all sorts of toxins, they can also become confused and attack your friendly and helpful thyroid cells as if they were some vile enemy, thus creating excessive inflammation.

2. **Hashimoto's is clinically revealed via one or both antibodies against the thyroid (anti-TPO, anti-Tg).** For a small minority, there are no antibodies at all, aka Seronegative Hashi's, which needs an ultrasound for diagnosis. Another small body may also have Graves' antibodies with their Hashi's—the hyperthyroid side of the coin. They can be TSI (Thyroid-stimulating immunoglobulins) and/

or TSAb (Thyroid-stimulating antibody), or the TRAb antibodies (thyroid stimulating hormone receptor).

3. **Hashimoto's falls under the umbrella term "Thyroiditis"** of which it's one of several varieties of autoimmune thyroid nuttiness, even if Hashi's is the most common.

4. **Hashimoto's may end up pairing with other non-thyroid autoimmune diseases, sooner or later.** Thus, the importance of controlling the attack, controlling inflammation, and being educated.

5. **Hashimoto's can make you sensitive to stress of any kind,** as well as to certain foods, infections, toxin exposure, certain supplements or medication, etc. Any of the latter might cause flare-ups like extra fatigue, pain, worsening gut symptoms, weakness, breathlessness, hair loss, etc. It's unique to you. Thus, the importance of being self-aware and proactive in responding to and/or treating what is going on.

6. **Many Hashi's patients end up needing thyroid medications.** Natural Desiccated Thyroid, or combining synthetic T3 with synthetic T4, have proven by many patients to be the most successful ways to treat one's hypothyroid state. But it's equally as important to get our free T3 and Free T4 "optimal", which seems to be a free T3 at the top part of the range, and a free T4 midrange. Both. To achieve the latter, without problems, iron and cortisol have to be good, too. Being on T3-only has worked for those with a very high Reverse T3—the latter an inactive thyroid hormone. T4-only is the most problematic medication, forcing the body to live for conversion alone to T3. It's not uncommon to see antibodies go up when starting NDT or T3. But patients report that ends when optimal or the use of that which will lower antibodies, like Low Dose Naltrexone.

7. **Genetic mutations are a strong underlying cause of Hashi-moto's, but environmental and gut triggers can play a role as well.** Often one sees different autoimmune diseases in family members, even if some do not.

8. **The antibodies attack caused by Hashimoto's disease can push your inflammation levels up,** which in turn causes more inflammation and problems.   And those same antibodies are slowly destroying your thyroid.

9. **Patients report that the majority of doctors are seriously uneducated about Hashimoto's disease,** thus why this book is important to help you be informed and proactive in your relationship with a doctor, or as your own best advocate.

10. **There are important and hopeful strategies via patient examples about putting Hashimoto's Thyroiditis into remission.** Remission means one lowers and stops the autoimmune attack, which in turn can lower symptoms and miseries. Sometimes "cure" is used in place of remission, but "remission" fits an autoimmune situation which could come back if strategies aren't continued to be implemented.

You will see the subject of all 10 points discussed throughout the book.

NOTES

Chapter 3

Hashimoto's disease: History and Stages

In 1912, a young, 30-year-old Japanese doctor and scientist wrote a distinguished paper for a German journal of clinical surgery called 'Archiv für Klinische Chirurgie" (which means Archive for Clinical Surgery for our non-German readers). His detailed paper was about a 'new' type of goiter (an enlargement of the thyroid gland). He called it "struma lymphomatosa".

His name was Hakaru Hashimoto, MD, PhD. He was associated with the medical school at Kyushu University in Japan. It's the 4th oldest University in Japan located in Fukuoka on the island of Kyushu.[1]

His "struma" means thyroid swelling, and "lymphomatous" refers to a large number of lymphocytes in the thyroid. Lymphocytes are a form of white blood cells used by the immune system to fight pathogens like

---

viruses, bacteria, fungus, and parasites—the bad guys.

Those "large" amounts of white blood cells which Dr. Hashimoto's observed turned out to be a big "ah-ha"! It was 1957 that the condition was finally connected to being an autoimmune disorder towards a specific gland—the unnatural attack of the thyroid by a copious amount of confused white blood cells called B cells[2] which are releasing all the Y-shaped antibodies[3].

> When there is no confusion, these Y-shaped antibodies will recognize bad guys in your body and attempt to neutralize them. When there is confusion, it's called an autoimmune disease.

Dr. Hashimoto's original term of "struma lymphomatous" remained the favored terminology in medical journals into the 1940s through the 1960s. Eventually, the condition of excess white blood cells attacking the thyroid was simply named Hashimoto's disease—a great honor for Dr. Hashimoto's. Though you will still see the term "struma lymphomatous" used in certain journal articles, it's now more common to see simply Hashimoto's disease or Hashimoto's Thyroiditis.

> Interesting to note that the initial patients which Dr. Hashimoto's studied between 1905 and 1909 were all women, underscoring that it happens to women far more than men, even if some men are still susceptible.[4]

---

[2] https://en.wikipedia.org/wiki/B_cell
[3] https://courses.lumenlearning.com/boundless-microbiology/chapter/antibodies/
[4] https://journals.lww.com/theendocrinologist/Citation/2001/03000/Hakaru_Hashimoto__1881_1934__and_His_Disease.1.aspx

The Rise of Hashimoto's Mentions

Cases of "struma lymphomatous"/Hashimoto's were now being identified in journals from the 1940s onward.[5]   And they were observing significant features on these kinds of thyroid glands:

- Some thyroid cells had become grainy, which are called Hürthle cells.
- The thyroids had lower iodine intake (thyroid hormones are composed of iodine) and thus lower production of thyroid hormones. They can also occur in goiters.
- Some of the thyroid cells were withering away and now smaller.
- Scaring and stiffness was seen in these thyroids.

It took 40 more years for literature to report that a major attack on enzymes in the thyroid called peroxidase (TPO) can occur.

 TAKE HEED: This sole mention of TPO is what has caused many doctors to fail to test a second identified Hashi's attack—towards thyroglobulin i.e. the anti-Tg, or anti-thyroglobulin. Thus, because one antibody can be high and another one not, some patients with Hashimoto's were, and are, being missed.

By 2013, it was concluded that Hashimoto's disease was now "considered the most prevalent autoimmune disease, as well as the most common endocrine disorder".[6][7]

---

[5] https://www.ncbi.nlm.nih.gov/pmc/articles/PMC3569966/
[6] https://www.ncbi.nlm.nih.gov/pubmed/23151083
[7] https://www.ncbi.nlm.nih.gov/books/NBK459262/

Stages of Hashimoto's Disease

Yes, it's possible to see certain general stages in the progress of Hashimoto's. Similar but different versions of stages have been proposed well by health entrepreneur Vedrana Högqvist Tabor[8] and pharmacist Isabella Wentz.[9]   Below represents stages of Hashimoto's as described by patients. And some stages can overlap!

Stage One:
The Calm Before the Storm: Predisposition

This stage represents an individual walking through life having a strong propensity, vulnerability, or risk in developing an autoimmune 'attack-the-thyroid' problem like Hashimoto's, but not necessarily being aware of any risk. Hashimoto's patients have also stated they were in this stage, watching other family members with Hashi's or other autoimmune issues, while they themselves had no clues of it going on in their own body…yet.

Length of time within this stage will vary. For some women, one can go decades in this predisposition stage to only finally see Hashi's reveal itself after menopause. Others may walk in this stage more briefly before seeing the manifestation of Hashimoto's, whether in childhood, teenage years, or adulthood. Far more women than men go through these stages, as well.

What is one particularly important component of this predisposition stage? Studies done of siblings[10] and families point strongly to a genetic vulnerability, i.e. inherited characteristics or conditions that can get passed down through generations. This

---

[8] https://medium.com/boosted/which-stage-of-hashimotos-are-you-in-14dfbefea1ae
[9] https://thyroidpharmacist.com/articles/5-stages-hashimotos-thyroiditis/
[10] https://www.ncbi.nlm.nih.gov/pmc/articles/PMC3271310/

genetic predisposition can also be triggered via various life triggers. This will be discussed in more detail in Chapter 4.

One German study[11] investigating "familial prevalence" found that the risk for developing autoimmune thyroid disease (AITD) "was 16-fold and 15-fold increased in children and siblings, respectively, of patients with AITD", especially for females. It also stated that "children and siblings of index cases with Hashimoto's thyroiditis had a 32-fold and 21-fold increased risk, respectively, for developing" Hashimoto's.

Stage Two:
The Rise of Antibodies—Silent for some,
Obvious for others

This stage is where one's over-reactive, misguided antibodies start to rise. Another *boooo! hiss!* In this stage, you may not be made aware of the discrete and nutty war being started in your body against your thyroid. Symptoms can be minor or none.

Rising antibodies revealed in this stage are one or both of two related to Hashimoto's disease. They are Thyroid Peroxidase Antibodies (anti-TPO or TPOAb) and Thyroglobulin antibodies (anti-thyroglobulin or TgAb).

Again, note that there are two thyroid antibodies shown above. Too many patients have reported their doctors only testing one of the two antibodies, usually the anti-peroxidase (anti-TPO). And that's a problem!

i.e. The one tested may be fine, thus you are told "You don't have Hashi's". But the one not tested, anti-thyroglobulin, may be high! Informed patients need to know what is going on with both, not just

---

[11] https://www.ncbi.nlm.nih.gov/pubmed/21287436

one. Even in the throes of Hashimoto's treatment, informed patients will test both to see their progress in bringing both down.

If you can catch the nutty war at this early 2nd stage, you might be able to reverse some damage by avoiding certain triggering foods like grains, dairy, sugar, etc., lowering stress in your life, treating inflammation, and other helpful supplements and more. When you get to Chapter 16, you'll see mentions of some of those patient-reported supplements.

There are different statistics as to what is the most common age when antibodies will start with this stage of onset. Some say ages 30-50.[12] Others say 40-60.[13] But even younger adults can start to see antibodies in this stage, just as post-menopausal women can be in this stage. Some children at different ages can also see the onset of Hashimoto's. The most common sex to see antibodies going up are female. But some males are susceptible, too, even if less common than females.

Stage Three:
The Growth and Onslaught of the Anti-Thyroid Army

This is the stage of growing symptoms and ballooning antibodies which are attacking the thyroid. Unfortunately, this is also the stage where a large body of those with Hashimoto's may finally catch the problem, though another percentage still don't realize it, nor are having the two antibodies tested by their doctors. All they know is "I have problems going on."

In this stage, you might notice a yin and yang of symptoms from your thyroid being attacked. One time, whether one day or many,

---

[12] https://en.wikipedia.org/wiki/Hashimoto%27s_thyroiditis
[13] Caturegli P, DeRemigis A, Rose NR. Hashimoto thyroiditis: clinical and diagnostic criteria. Autoimmunity Reviews. 2014;13(4-5):391–397.

you can feel very sluggish and hypothyroid. Then another time, you can have hyper-like symptoms such as palpitations, faster heart rate, anxiety, weight loss. The sluggish hypo symptoms are due to the failing thyroid; the hyper-like symptoms are due to the die off of thyroid hormones dumping into your cells.

> Ever been told you were bipolar
> (a mental health disorder)? That can happen when a doctor
> doesn't understand the yin and yang symptoms of an attacked
> thyroid, i.e. hypo to hyper, back and forth.

Here are other symptoms one may start to notice in this stage:
- easy fatigue
- poor stamina
- the need to nap
- digestive issues
- hair loss
- dry hair or skin
- feeling colder than you used to
- constipation
- depression
- rising blood pressure
- rising cholesterol
- delayed menstrual periods; heavier flow
- difficulty getting pregnant
- joint pain
- easy weight gain
- difficulty losing
- anxiety

This can also be the stage that you might notice a lump on your neck where the thyroid is. Or you might notice difficulty swallowing or discomfort wearing a turtleneck shirt. You might feel more reactions to certain foods you eat, or to stress.

With lab work, one might notice the free T3 and free T4 being lower in the range than they should be. Healthy levels seem to always put both right above midrange, patients have noticed in others.[14]

Unfortunately, in Stages 2 or 3, one might be seeing a doctor who tells you something similar to "let it run its course" or "wait it out". Informed Hashi's patients feel that is akin to stating *"Just continue to go through the miserable symptoms of the attack which could get worse!"*

And going through this stage can predispose some patients to developing a cortisol problem due to the chronic stress of the attack. It's not fun having either too-low or too-high cortisol. You'll learn more about adrenals and cortisol when you get to Chapter 11.

Stage Four:
Fighting Back with Treatment Strategies

This is an important stage in fighting back at what's going on. Fighting back may have started in an earlier stage, but definitely should continue now. That is contrary to what some patients have reported that their doctor said to them, i.e. "Just let it run its course".

This stage involves a variety of treatments you can implement to stop the attack and feel better. Once you get there, Chapters 9, 10, 11, 13 and especially 16, cover issues and treatment to stop the attack.

---

[14] http://stopthethyroidmadness.com/lab-values

Stage Five:

A Commitment to Life-long Management

Can you stop everything you've done to lower the antibodies and feel better for the rest of your life? Apparently not.

When patients have tried to reintroduce certain triggering foods, back came the rise of the antibodies. When patients tried to lower or stop their thyroid medications (after their thyroid was somewhat destroyed by the attack), back came a too-low free T3 and free T4, and back came hypothyroid symptoms.

Granted, there are some autoimmune diets that once implemented, patients have been able to reintroduce some foods without problems. But other foods may not work well if you try them once again. Gluten can be an example, as can foods that cause an allergic reaction.

This is a life-long management of your Hashimoto's and autoimmune tendencies which can entail changing the way you eat, keeping your gut healthy, lowering stress, keeping your immune system in good shape as best as you can by avoiding triggers, and for some, steering clear of triggering chemical exposure.

Hashimoto's and Rise of Other Autoimmune Conditions, aka Pairing

Yes, there are a certain body of Hashimoto's patients who deal with other autoimmune issues, as well, such as rheumatoid arthritis, type 1 diabetes, multiple sclerosis (MS), lupus or even pernicious anemia. You will learn about other autoimmune issues in Chapter 7—the dysfunctional family.

Ever heard the term Hashitoxicosis?[15]

This is a condition of having both Hashi's antibodies (anti-TPO, anti-Thyroglobulin) plus having Graves' antibodies (such as TRAb, aka TSAb or TBII antibodies). And it's pretty miserable, report patients who found themselves in those autoimmune shoes. Low Dose Naltrexone is a favored way to treat it, say patients.

TIDBITS

■ For some who get Hashimoto's,
   their first sign is weight loss.

[15] https://www.hindawi.com/journals/crie/2016/6210493/

NOTES

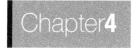 **Genetics and Environmental Triggers for** Hashimoto's disease

Part One: The Genetic Trigger

In 2017, a study was done to document the occurrence of Hashimoto's among family members.[16] The study found that 46% of the 264 patients with Hashimoto's disease included in the study had at least one relative with the same.

Among first degree relatives, meaning parents, siblings, or children, the risk of developing Hashi's was stated to be 9-fold higher as compared to the "general population". Specifically, "parents and siblings each had a 6-fold higher risk, while children had a 3-fold higher risk" of having Hashimoto's.

We also can see that several studies show the risk of Hashimoto's increasing with age.

---

[16] https://www.ncbi.nlm.nih.gov/pubmed/28273382

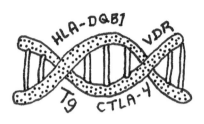

All the latter seems to strongly imply that certain genetic variations can play a strong role in the development of an autoimmune thyroid problem, i.e. some variations make you "vulnerable".

Have you done genetic testing? It doesn't appear to be one gene that influences the development of Hashimoto's, but several genes and their variants.

Examples of genes involved in Hashimoto's disease

1. Human Leukocyte Antigen (HLA)

This is a set of genes which, when working correctly, help your immune system differentiate between:

a) proteins made by the bad guys (bacteria and viruses), vs

b) those made by your own body.

Thus, if there is a mutation/variation on an HLA gene, your immune system may not be getting the right message and can become confused as to what's an enemy and what is not![17] One gene identified as a possibility within this complex is called **HLA-DQB1**[18]. Another gene identified as possibly linked to Hashimoto's if a variant occurs is called **HLA-DR3**.

2. Vitamin D Receptor (VDR)

It appears that if a mutation of this gene causes less production of Vitamin D, one can become more susceptible to Hashimoto's.[19] [20]

---

[17] https://www.endocrine-abstracts.org/ea/0037/ea0037gp.26.10
[18] https://ghr.nlm.nih.gov/gene/HLA-DQB1
[19] https://www.ncbi.nlm.nih.gov/pubmed/16721822/
[20] https://www.ncbi.nlm.nih.gov/pubmed/27468766

3. Thyroglobulin (Tg)

This thyroid gene provides instructions in making the thyroglobulin protein—the latter which when combined with iodine, makes thyroid hormones.[21] Problems in this gene may be associated with Hashi's[22], just as four particular mutations of this gene may be making your thyroid more susceptible to being attacked.[23] [24]

4. Cytotoxic T Lymphocyte Antigen-4 gene (CTLA-4)

This is a protein receptor gene which, when working correctly without variants, would down regulate your immune responses. Having a variant in this gene is not only implicated in Hashimoto's, but can predispose one to other autoimmune conditions like Graves', lupus and more.[25]

5. Protein Tyrosine Phosphatase Nonreceptor-Type 22 gene (PTPN22)

This gene, when working properly, is another regulator to promote immune stability. So, when it has a variant, it is a strong risk for Hashimoto's and other autoimmune diseases like rheumatoid arthritis.[26]

6. Cytokine Inflammation Genes

Turns out that mutations in various inflammation-related genes could predispose you to Hashimoto's and other autoimmune conditions.[27] Other related genes include chemokines, COX-2, IL-1a,

---

[21] https://ghr.nlm.nih.gov/gene/TG
[22] https://www.ncbi.nlm.nih.gov/pubmed/28942902
[23] https://www.ncbi.nlm.nih.gov/pmc/articles/PMC299918/
[24] https://www.ncbi.nlm.nih.gov/pmc/articles/PMC3960735/
[25] https://en.wikipedia.org/wiki/CTLA-4
[26] https://www.nature.com/articles/nrrheum.2014.109
[27] https://www.ncbi.nlm.nih.gov/pubmed/17115419

IL-1b, IL-6, IL-8, IL-18, MMP-9, 5-LOX, and VEGF.[28]

7. Protein Tyrosine Phosphatase Nonreceptor-Type 22 (PTPN22) Gene

This gene provides instructions for making a particular protein and regulates immune cells called T cells. There are studies which imply it could be implicated in Hashimoto's if a variant exists.[29] [30]

When it comes to gene mutations, though, it's all about risk, not definite probability.

Part Two: Environmental Triggers

There are a slew of research articles pointing to this second significant factor influencing Hashimoto's disease, whether simply bringing on one's genetic propensity for Hashimoto's thyroiditis, or making existing Hashi's worse.

The following list represents those environmental risks. Remember that risk means "potential". None of these listed risks means you will categorically have problems because of them. But with one's genetics, the risk of these causing problems is increased, making each of these worthy of understanding and keeping an eye on.

List of Environment Triggers

- **Chronic infections** In autoimmune-susceptible individuals, a pathogen which would result in a normal autoimmune response by the body, may go overboard and start attacking healthy

---

[28] https://www.ncbi.nlm.nih.gov/pmc/articles/PMC3271310/

[29] https://www.ncbi.nlm.nih.gov/pubmed/20615141

[30] https://www.semanticscholar.org/paper/The-protein-tyrosine-phosphatase-non-receptor-type-Dultz-Matheis/4f3d79fd82bed3844e4134abb8ff6d07aa1d6ba7

tissue. Or, damage caused by a normal and healthy immune response may be seen as another enemy by your overreactive immune system.[31] For example, strong immune responses to Lyme disease and the herpes virus have even been shown to initiate an autoimmune reaction in some patients.

- **Changes in sex hormones** Especially in females, fluctuations in sex hormones might trigger one's overreactive immune response and thus the onset of Hashi's.[32][33] This might occur in puberty, pregnancy or menopause…with the latter appearing to be the biggest risk based on patient reports.

- **Iodine supplementation** On the positive side, contrary to the naysaying and scare-mongering you will read, iodine supplementation in reasonable amounts (as compared to too-high amounts) has been cited by many Hashi's patients as the reason their antibodies came down. That is huge and was reported on the Stop the Thyroid Madness website and books years ago. Others have used iodine successfully to shrink thyroid nodules along with the use of natural desiccated thyroid or T3. But as experienced by some susceptible individuals, iodine supplementation has made their antibodies go up. This is why you need to be familiar with "companion nutrients", as coined by author Lynne Farrow who wrote *The Iodine Crisis: What You Don't Know about Iodine Can Wreck Your Life*. These nutrients help prepare for the toxin release of bromides, chlorides and other halides—the latter which can raise antibodies. The Stop the Thyroid Madness website has an important page about those companion nutrients.[34] And once started on iodine, it can be about "going slow, staying low", not amounts greater than you might need or which can

[31] https://www.ncbi.nlm.nih.gov/pmc/articles/PMC2665673/
[32] https://www.ncbi.nlm.nih.gov/pmc/articles/PMC6119719/
[33] https://www.sciencedirect.com/science/article/abs/pii/S1568997211002941
[34] https://stopthethyroidmadness.com/2013/12/29/companion-nutrients-the-key-to-iodine-protocol/

raise the risk of flares. For example, some do fine as high as 50 mg, but there are many who do better staying much lower.

- **Pesticide exposure** This can include most chemicals used to control harmful insects on plants, as well as against rodents. Also included are sprays used to prevent fungus, bacteria and larvae. There is evidence that the chemical in these sprays, which nearly all of us can be exposed to, can trigger an overreactive autoimmune response.[35]

- **Toxin exposure** This area can include exposure to high heavy metals, cleaning supply chemicals, what we breathe, exposures where we work. Detoxing any of these substances can also increase exposure due to the internal movement of the detox. They all can potentially cause an overreaction by one's immune system.[36]

- **Excessive radiation therapy** Radiation is often used in the treatment of cancers. This can also include the radioactive material from a nuclear fallout or nuclear accidents like Chernobyl[37]. The radiation itself can trigger an excess immune response.[38]

- **Low Vitamin D levels** Deficient levels of vitamin D are implicated in those with Hashimoto's, whether from genetic variations or seeing a drop from being on T4-only medications (or underdosed on better thyroid meds due to a doctor's over-reliance on the lousy TSH lab test). In fact, research found that up to 82% of Hashi's patients had low vitamin D.[39] That's a high percentage! What is optimal? Opinions are all over the map. But the Vitamin D council reports having a blood result of at least 50. Others shoot for the 60-80 range.

---

[35] https://blumhealthmd.com/2018/06/28/the-link-between-pesticides-and-hashimotos/
[36] https://www.mindbodygreen.com/0-12346/11-everyday-toxins-that-are-harming-your-thyroid.html
[37] https://www.ncbi.nlm.nih.gov/pubmed/9737280
[38] https://stanfordhealthcare.org/medical-treatments/r/radiation-therapy/about-this-treatment/conditions-treated.html
[39] https://www.holtorfmed.com/vitamin-d-autoimmune-thyroid-disease/

- **Deficient Selenium levels**   Numerous patient reports over the years, which Stop the Thyroid Madness website and books focus on, have found that taking selenium, 200-400 mcg, does a great job lowering the high anti-TPO levels! And research[40] does show that low levels contributes to Hashi's antibodies. This is why selenium supplementation is included as one of several companion nutrients[41] to prepare for iodine use. But... patients found it wise to test selenium first to make sure it's not too high due to a methylation problem.[42] A methylation problem means it's not breaking down for use.

- **Certain anti-cancer medications like cytokines, interferon, and tyrosine kinase inhibitors**[43] [44] Yes, the side effects of some anti-cancer medications can raise the risk of pushing one into Hashimoto's disease.

- **Certain Multiple Sclerosis medications**[45] The medication in particular is called alemtuzumab and has the potential side effect of an autoimmune response.

- **Cold weather exposure**[46]   Study showed that women living in Siberia showed a high prevalence of thyroid peroxidase (TPO) antibodies. Brrrrrrr.

- **Smoking** This risk in causing an autoimmune reaction may be due to the negative charged ion 'thiocyanate' which is generated when smoking.[47]

- **Triclosan in antibacterial soaps** If you have some anti-bacterial soaps laying around, know that there are many studies[48]

---

[40] https://academic.oup.com/jcem/article/87/4/1687/2374966
[41] https://stopthethyroidmadness.com/2013/12/29/companion-nutrients-the-key-to-iodine-protocol/
[42] http://stopthethyroidmadness.com/selenium
[43] https://www.ncbi.nlm.nih.gov/pmc/articles/PMC5053048/
[44] https://www.ncbi.nlm.nih.gov/pubmed/23750887
[45] https://www.ncbi.nlm.nih.gov/pmc/articles/PMC5971042/
[46] https://www.ncbi.nlm.nih.gov/pubmed/21732471
[47] https://www.ncbi.nlm.nih.gov/pubmed/8957745
[48] https://www.science.gov/topicpages/t/triclosan+modulates+thyroid.html

implicating triclosan in causing thyroid problems. So, there is supposition that it may contribute to Hashimoto's as well.

- **Soy** There is one particular study[49] showing a correlation between drinking soy milk and the rise of Hashimoto's.

- **Living near petrochemical complexes** I personally used to live near a large petrochemical complex. And though I didn't get Hashi's from that exposure, this caught my eye.[50]

- **The trigger of being female** Percentages vary, but it's clear than females are far more likely to develop Hashimoto's disease than men, as well as other autoimmune diseases.[51][52]

- **Epstein Barr Virus** Research, as well as a certain body of reported experiences, show that it's mostly the other way around i.e. the stress of Hashimoto's thyroiditis causing one to have reactivated EBV. Or, the stress of being hypothyroid or poorly treated, on top of other life stresses, activating latent EBV. The inflammation caused by an EBV infection could promote an increase in cytokine proteins which could signal an autoimmune overactivity.[53]

- **Lack of childhood exposure to microbes** It's proposed that children who weren't exposed to microbes (aka lived a bit too clean, didn't play much outdoors or in the dirt) can have a high risk of autoimmune diseases later. Makes you wonder about today's children who may not be encouraged to put the electronics down and go outside and play.[54]

- **Chronic Hepatitis C Virus** It appears that autoimmune diseases

---

[49] https://www.researchgate.net/publication/282980278_A_case_report_Soy_milk_-_a_possible_cause_of_Hashimoto's_thyroiditis
[50] https://www.ncbi.nlm.nih.gov/pubmed/19913221
[51] https://www.sciencedirect.com/science/article/pii/S0091302214000466#b0600
[52] https://www.ncbi.nlm.nih.gov/pubmed/24793874
[53] https://www.ncbi.nlm.nih.gov/pubmed/25931043
[54] https://www.ncbi.nlm.nih.gov/pubmed/23127244

like Hashimoto's are common with those who have untreated hepatitis C virus.[55] Hepatitis C is an inflammation disease of the liver. It's often contacted via the infectious blood or fluids in another person.

Chapters 9 and 10 will cover important gut triggers for you to be aware of.

TIDBITS

- Did you know that working out too hard in a gym can contribute as a trigger in making Hashimoto's worse? Stress is stress.

- Many Hashimoto's patients report that getting sick seems to cause their disease to flare, and/or they feel worse than others seem to feel and/or can take longer to recover.

- Be careful with that room freshener spray. They are known to have carcinogens and toxins that you may want to avoid breathing constantly.

---

[55] https://www.ncbi.nlm.nih.gov/pmc/articles/PMC4716530/

NOTES

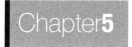

Chapter 5

Interesting Research and Statistics about Hashimoto's

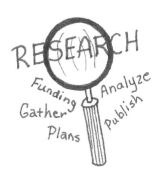

Ever heard of King Nebuchadnezzar? Not only is he mentioned in the Old Testament, ruling from 605 BC to 562 BC, he was involved in the first recorded incident of doing a clinical trial, aka research[56].

He had one group eating nothing but wine and meat, and the other group nothing but beans and water. And those who just ate the beans and water appeared healthier than the former group.

All these years later, we have plenty of interesting research concerning Autoimmune Hashimoto's disease. Plus, you will see many research articles posted as footnotes in each chapter.

---

[56] https://www.ncbi.nlm.nih.gov/pmc/articles/PMC2612069/

Here are 46 short summaries of what is contained in research and related articles about Hashimoto's.

1. The **female-to-male ratio for Hashimoto's is at least 10:1**
    https://www.ncbi.nlm.nih.gov/books/NBK459262/

2. **The pathology of Hashi's is diagnosed five to ten times more often in women than men, and its incidence increases with age (the peak of the number of cases is between 45 and 65); however, it can also be diagnosed in children.** https://www.hindawi.com/
    journals/jir/2015/979167/abs/

3. **Most women are diagnosed between the ages of 30 to 50 years old.** https://www.ncbi.nlm.nih.gov/books/NBK459262/

4. **The most common antibody is anti-thyroid peroxidase (anti-TPO). Many also form thyroglobulin antibodies (anti-Tg) and a smaller body have the TSH receptor blocking antibodies (TBII). There is a small subset of the population, no more than 10% with the clinically evident disease, that are serum antibody-negative.** https://www.ncbi.nlm.nih.gov/books/NBK459262/

5. **After age six, Hashimoto's is the most common cause of hypothyroidism in the United States and in those areas of the world where iodine intake is inadequate.** https://www.ncbi.nlm.
    nih.gov/books/NBK459262/

6. **The incidence of Hashimoto's is estimated at 3.5 per 1000 per year in women and 0.8 per 1000 per year in men.** https://www.
    ncbi.nlm.nih.gov/books/NBK459262/

7. **Twin studies have shown an increased concordance of auto-immune thyroiditis in monozygotic twins (from the same egg; identical) as compared with dizygotic twins (from two eggs; not identical). Danish studies have demonstrated**

concordance rates of 55% in monozygotic twins, compared with only 3% in dizygotic twins. https://www.ncbi.nlm.nih.gov/books/NBK459262/

8. Data suggests that 79% of predisposition is due to genetic factors, allotting 21% for environmental and sex hormone influences. https://www.ncbi.nlm.nih.gov/books/NBK459262/

9. Hashimoto's thyroiditis (HT) is one of the most frequent autoimmune diseases and has been reported to be associated with gastric disorders in 10% to 40% of patients. https://www.ncbi.nlm.nih.gov/books/NBK459262/

10. About 40% of patients with autoimmune gastritis also present with Hashimoto's thyroiditis. Chronic autoimmune gastritis leads to impairment of hydrochloric acid and intrinsic factor production. The patients go on to develop hypochlorhydria-dependent iron-deficient anemia, leading to pernicious anemia, and severe gastric atrophy. https://www.ncbi.nlm.nih.gov/books/NBK459262/

11. You are more likely to develop Hashimoto's disease if you have other autoimmune disorders from the autoimmune family. https://www.niddk.nih.gov/health-information/endocrine-diseases/hashimotos-disease

12. Inadequate Vitamin D levels are strongly associated with Hashimoto's (whether causing an onset or with active Hashi's) https://www.ncbi.nlm.nih.gov/pmc/articles/PMC5244647/

13. Supplementing with Vitamin D in Hashi's patients with low Vit. D levels can help lower antibodies in some. https://www.ncbi.nlm.nih.gov/pmc/articles/PMC5244647/

14. Anti-TPO levels were significantly higher in 186 out of 218 vitamin D deficient Hashi's patients compared to 32 out of

186 Hashi's patients with no vitamin D deficiency http://www. nuclmed.gr/magazine/eng/sept15/07.pdf

15. There is evidence that the genesis and progression of autoimmune thyroid disorders (Hashimoto's) may be significantly affected from a changing intestinal microbial composition or even from overt dysbiosis. https://link.springer. com/article/10.1007/s11154-018-9467-y

16. Hashimoto's patients have altered gut microbiota i.e. abundant levels of Blautia, Roseburia, Ruminococcus torque group, Romboutsia, Dorea, Fusicatenibacter, and Eubacterium. Hallii group genera were increased, whereas the abundance levels of Fecalibacterium, Bacteroides, Prevotella 9, and Lachnoclostridium genera were decreased. https://www.liebert pub.com/doi/abs/10.1089/thy.2017.0395

17. In just the US, Hashimoto's thyroiditis (HT) affects more than 14 million individuals in the United States, most of them women. http://tinyurl.com/y5thypu6

18. Thyroid replacement therapy has long been the foundation of medical treatment for HT; however, recent research supports a role for nutritional approaches (2018) http://tinyurl.com/ y5thypu6

19. The frequency of Hashimoto's disease is a growing trend. Among Caucasians, it is estimated at approximately 5%. https:// www.hindawi.com/journals/jir/2015/979167/abs/

20. There can be an association between Hashi's and Papillary Thyroid Cancer and between Hashi's and Thyroid Lymphoma. No association was found between Hashi's and follicular, medullary, or anaplastic thyroid cancer. https://www.frontiersin. org/articles/10.3389/fonc.2017.00053/full

21. In Hashimoto's, oxidant status ("free radicals," which can cause damage) is increased and antioxidant status is decreased in Hashimoto's. https://eje.bioscientifica.com/view/journals/ eje/173/6/ 791.xml

22. Though very rare, some patients with Hashimoto's disease can experience neck pain. https://link.springer.com/article/10.1007/ s40618-017-0655-5

23. The presence of Hashimoto's antithyroid antibodies is associated with a 200% to 300% increase of miscarriage. https://search.proquest.com/openview/02d8eeedd2496926b9efc078 400f28a5/1?pq-origsite=gscholar&cbl=32528

24. Fructose or lactose malabsorption was present in 73.3% of Hashi's patients, as well as gastrointestinal symptoms. https:// www.nature.com/articles/ejcn2015167

25. Patients who have higher anti-TPO and anti-Tg levels have significantly lower quality of life domain scores. https://www. sciencedirect.com/science/article/pii/S1607551X16301152

26. A number of environmental factors like viral infection, smoking, stress & iodine intake are associated with the progression of Hashimoto's and even Graves' disease. https:// www.ncbi.nlm.nih.gov/pubmed/23105486

27. Multiple Autoimmune Syndrome (MAS) is the name for those with at least three autoimmune diseases. https://www.ncbi. nlm.nih.gov/pmc/articles/PMC3150011/

28. Low-level laser therapy (LLLT) may have promising results in improving the thyroid gland in Hashimoto's patients and decreasing antibodies. More research is needed. https://www. hindawi.com/journals/ije/2018/8387530/

29. **How Inositol and selenium help lower antibodies and can return a Hashimoto's patient to a non-symptom state.** https://www.ncbi.nlm.nih.gov/pmc/articles/PMC5331475/

30. **Though there is controversy in research as to whether low Vitamin D levels actually promote Hashimoto's** https://journals.aace.com/doi/abs/10.4158/EP15934.OR, **there is other research that shows how having good Vitamin K levels helps lower hardening of the arteries as well as prevents high blood pressure** https://www.ncbi.nlm.nih.gov/pubmed/28396533. **(Patients frequently take vitamin K2 with their vitamin D3 supplementation).**

31. **Vitamin K2 is not only a major player in bone health, but it also keeps calcium from accumulating in the walls of blood vessels.** https://www.ncbi.nlm.nih.gov/pmc/articles/PMC4566462/

32. **Common variants in PDE10A and MAF gene regions may influence whether patients develop Graves' disease or Hashimoto's disease.** https://www.ncbi.nlm.nih.gov/pubmed/25683181

33. **A disruption in the amount of good gut bacteria can result in depression or anxiety.** https://www.nature.com/articles/mp201650

34. **Caffeine may have the potential to be an effective anti-microbial agent against some species of bad bacteria.** https://jbs.camden.rutgers.edu/Gaula_Donegan_caffeine

35. **Antibiotic use will strongly alter one's gut bacteria and thus can cause depression, anxiety.** https://www.ncbi.nlm.nih.gov/pubmed/26580313

36. **A diverse gut bacteria is highly important to teach your**

immune system to do an appropriate job. https://www.ncbi.nlm. nih.gov/pmc/articles/PMC4143175/

37. **Conversely, an abnormal amount of gut bacteria can make one's immune system mess up.** https://www.ncbi.nlm.nih.gov/ pubmed/29367525

38. **The prevalence of Celiac in children with Hashimoto's is higher than in children without Hashimoto's.** https://www.ncbi. nlm.nih.gov/pmc/articles/PMC4959737/

39. **Pregnancy does not appear to be a trigger for Hashimoto's.** https://www.ncbi.nlm.nih.gov/pubmed/9789594

40. **Lupus patients are twice as likely to acquire Hashimoto's disease.** https://www.ncbi.nlm.nih.gov/pubmed/28544477

41. **Low vitamin D may play a role in children and Hashimoto's.** https://www.ncbi.nlm.nih.gov/pubmed/22876540

42. **Pituitary antibodies are more common in Hashimoto's thyroiditis and suggest that they appear late during its natural history.** https://www.ncbi.nlm.nih.gov/pmc/articles/ PMC3338955/?tool=pmcentrez

43. **ATDs (Autoimmune Thyroid Diseases) are associated with abnormalities of glucose metabolism and thus increased risk of developing diabetes mellitus type 1 and type 2.** https://www. science.gov/topicpages/h/hashimoto+disease#

44. **Nutrient deficiencies usually observed in patients suffering from ATD are: protein deficiencies, vitamin deficiencies (A, C, B6, B5, B1) and mineral deficiencies (phosphorus, magnesium, potassium, sodium, chromium). Proper diet helps to reduce the symptoms of the disease, maintains a healthy weight and prevents the occurrence of malnutrition.** https://www.science.gov/topicpages/h/hashimoto+disease#

45. **Unhealthy changes in one's gut bacteria is an important trigger in the development of autoimmune disease like Hashimoto's and other similar diseases.** https://clinicaltrials.gov/ct2/show/NCT03390582

46. **PCOS may be a kind of autoimmune disease and has close association with AIT (autoimmune thyroid)** https://www.ncbi.nlm.nih.gov/pmc/articles/PMC3832324/

All the latter is nowhere near an exhaustive list of interesting info in research and studies about Hashimoto's, but does give you a great taste.

NOTES

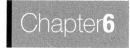

Thyroiditis: The Umbrella over Hashimoto's and Other Autoimmune Thyroid Disorders

Many times, in serious articles or research, you'll see Hashimoto's described as "Hashimoto's Thyroiditis".

What in the world is Thyroiditis?

It's a group of organ-specific, immune system disorders of the thyroid under the same umbrella, of which Hashi's is the most common version in the group. They all involve an unnatural attack of the thyroid gland with the abnormal purpose to destroy and defeat. And they all result in inflammation of the thyroid, even if the order of actions can be a bit different. Some attack results are slow; others are quite fast.

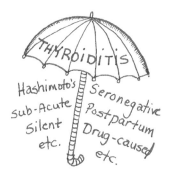

Another term you might see in literature is the diagnosis of Autoimmune thyroid disease (AITD). Though the term includes all the different Thyroiditis disorders I list next, it also includes Graves' disease, the autoimmune disorder that causes hyperthyroidism.

Below is my mother at age 20, skinny from her Graves' disease, one of the diseases under the term Autoimmune thyroid disease (AITD). But some Graves' patients may also have Hashimoto's antibodies, as well.

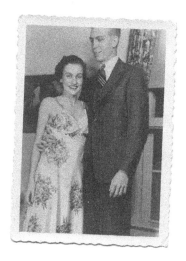

Most of the time in their use in literature, "Thyroiditis" and "Autoimmune Thyroid Disease" are referring to the same thing—an immune system nuttiness specific to the thyroid, even if Graves' isn't under Thyroiditis but under AITD. In this chapter, I'll stick with the word "thyroiditis" so you can learn about those conditions similar to, but different from, Hashimoto's.

Next are most common forms of Thyroiditis. Symptoms can be similar i.e. one can have hyper-like symptoms from the attack like anxiety, nervousness, high heart rate, palpitations, heat intolerance, etc., then end up with hypothyroid type symptoms, including fatigue, weight gain, hair loss, depression, concentration problems, swelling and more.

Hashimoto's Disease

Hashimoto's Disease, aka Hashi's and which is the main focus of this book, is the most common form of thyroiditis and the most common form of hypothyroidism. Antibodies are present, showing an attack on your thyroid, whether anti-TPO or anti-thyroglobulin or both. Genetic variations/mutations are a strong underlying cause, and there are environmental factors which can either bring on Hashi's, or make it worse.

Seronegative Thyroiditis, also called Seronegative Autoimmune Thyroiditis (seronegative CAT)

This is considered a milder, less aggressive form of Hashimoto's and often without serum antibodies, which is why an ultrasound might be needed to firmly diagnosis Seronegative. Cells in the thyroid might show antibodies, even if blood will not. Seronegative thyroiditis might also result in a goiter. For some, this might be the same as De Quervain's below. Literature states that anywhere from 5-10% of patients with Hashi's have the Seronegative form.

Subacute Thyroiditis, also called De Quervain's Thyroiditis

This form of thyroiditis was remarkably discovered in 1904[57]—eight years before Hashimoto's. It will have no antibodies and can involve inflammation and pain of the gland and a quick release of excess thyroid in your blood. Some feel it's caused by a virus of the thyroid, and can occur after one has had an upper respiratory tract viral infection. Pain of the thyroid is common, even though De Quervain's is considered sub-acute as a whole. Some have fever. Taking aspirin to reduce inflammation, plus bed rest, is recommended by doctors. Patients can recover from this.

---

[57] https://en.wikipedia.org/wiki/De_Quervain%27s_thyroiditis

Postpartum Thyroiditis

This form of post-birth thyroiditis is common, and may play a role in post-partum depression. Antibodies will be present and you may have no pain in the thyroid at all. It will start out with symptoms of hyperthyroidism, including a fast heart rate, easy weight loss, feeling nervous, tired, and not liking heat. It will move into hypothyroidism, and some women will remain hypothyroid the rest of their lives, while others will have a remission. Cause is not always known. It's stated that one in five women will have it again with a new birth.[58]

Silent Thyroiditis, also called Silent Lymphocytic Thyroiditis

This condition is similar to postpartum thyroiditis above, but can be more sporadic and not necessarily after a baby is born. It does not usually have pain of the thyroid, i.e. "silent". For some, it is recoverable within a few months, though others may have lifelong hypo. Cause is generally unknown.

Drug-caused Thyroiditis

The following drugs are said to promote thyroiditis. They can also just interfere with thyroid function and make one more hypothyroid. Examples are:

- *amiodarone*[59]: used in the treatment of tachyarrhythmias aka tachycardia of the heart and can raise RT3 and lower Free T3.
- *interferon-alpha therapy*[60]: used to treat chronic hepatitis C virus and may produce thyroid antibodies
- *lithium*[61]: used in higher amounts for the treatment of bipolar disorders, mania, and unipolar and bipolar depression.

---

[58] https://www.thyroid.org/postpartum-thyroiditis/
[59] https://www.ncbi.nlm.nih.gov/pubmed/11294826
[60] https://www.ncbi.nlm.nih.gov/pubmed/11250770
[61] https://www.ncbi.nlm.nih.gov/pmc/articles/PMC3568739/

The following are often shown in lists as promoting an autoimmune attack on the thyroid, but research is not at all conclusive about these causing that problem.

- *nitroprusside:* Used to treat high blood pressure and in fact, can help thyroid function during heart bypass surgery.
- *perchlorate:* Can block iodine uptake into the thyroid gland.
- *sulfonylureas:* Used to lower high blood glucose levels. Old research implies anti-thyroid, but nothing about autoimmune effects.
- *thalidomide:* A cancer drug which may mess up thyroid function, but research is weak that it would cause an autoimmune thyroid issue

Radiation Induced Thyroiditis

This rare condition can occur after the use of radiation treatment to treat hyperthyroidism, or radiation used to treat head or neck cancer. Pain is common. It can result in lifelong hypothyroidism. No antibodies are present.

Acute Thyroiditis

Also called Suppurative thyroiditis, this is caused by a bacterial or other infection in the thyroid, which is very rare. It can go away with treatment of the initial infection. No antibodies are present.

Riedel's Thyroiditis

A rare version of thyroiditis, this is about dense fibrosis in the thyroid causing inflammation, and this may be more of a fibroid disease. With this, you can also have hypoparathyroidism, hoarseness from problems to your larynx, and a compression of your tracheal tube. Your thyroid will feel quite hard.

Ord's Thyroiditis / Atrophic thyroiditis

This was first mentioned by Dr. William Miller Ord in 1877.   This form of thyroiditis refers to a reduced thyroid size, and is basically very similar to Hashimoto's, i.e. one or both antibodies will be attacking the thyroid. It's more common in European countries. Ord's/Atrophic Thyroiditis patients tend to see their thyroid atrophy, meaning shrink down, rather than form an enlarged goiter.

Hashimoto's Encephalopathy

There's a condition called Hashimoto's encephalopathy (HE)[62] which can occur to a very tiny minority of Hashimoto's patients. And though it's rare, it's important to know about it.

Affecting the brain and the way it functions, HE has symptoms which vary between individuals, such as confusion, memory problems, disorientation, seizures, difficulty walking, muscle jerking, trouble with speech plus irritability. In the worst of cases, delusions and hallucinations.

Most literature states that the cause is unknown, other than being associated with Hashimoto's. Treatment often involves the use of a strong corticosteroid like prednisone or Medrol, i.e. it's treatable! If you have this, talk to your doctor about the best treatment.

◆ ◆ ◆

Some of the above was borrowed from the Thyroiditis page on the patient-to-patient website Stop the Thyroid Madness. More has been added above. *https://stopthethyroidmadness.com/thyroiditis/*

---

[62] https://rarediseases.info.nih.gov/diseases/8570/hashimoto-encephalopathy

NOTES

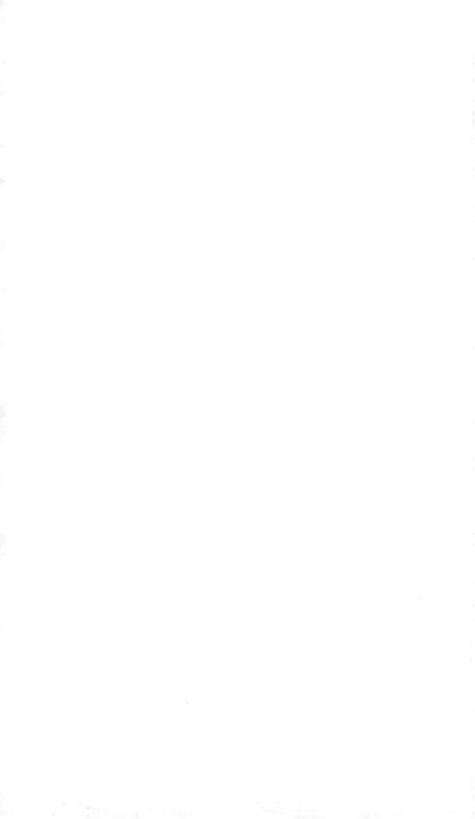

Chapter 7

Hashimoto's and the Dysfunctional Family of Autoimmune Issues

As an autoimmune disease, Hashimoto's disease is part of a large dysfunctional family of confused immune system diseases, attacking your own tissues or glands. So, if you have Hashi's, you have autoimmune overreaction "company".

Here's a list of some of the more well-known members in the dysfunctional autoimmune disease family:

Addison's disease: attack of the adrenal glands and causes seriously low cortisol, causing lifelong cortisol supplementation. President John F. Kennedy in the United States had Addison's, as did author Jane Austen in England.

Alopecia areata: causes hair loss on the scalp and sometimes other areas of the body. Sometimes doctors mistakenly use this term to describe hair loss due to low iron or hypothyroidism. Not the same.

Celiac disease: immune attack in the small intestine in response to gluten; damages the villi and inhibits nutrient absorption. Patients have to find out if they simply have gluten intolerance, also called Non-Celiac Gluten Sensitivity (NCGS), or Celiac.

Crohn's disease: inflammatory bowel disease (IBD); can cause abdominal pain, severe diarrhea, fatigue, malnutrition

Diabetes type 1: immune system attack on pancreatic cells that produce insulin

Gastritis (Autoimmune atrophic): immune system destruction of certain cells that line the stomach

Guillain-barre Syndrome: an immune system attack of one's nerves, causing weakness and tingling

Graves' disease: attack of the thyroid causing hyperthyroidism

Graves' ophthalmopathy: attack of eye muscles and other ocular tissues

Hashimoto's Encephalopathy: rare condition associated with Hashimoto's that negatively affects the brain

Hashimoto's Thyroiditis: immune system attack on the thyroid

Inflammatory Bowel Disease (IBD): related to immune attack of virus, bacteria, or food, leading to bowel injury and diarrhea

Lupus: can cause a facial rash, fatigue, joint and muscle pain and an attack of organs

Multiple sclerosis (MS): an immune system response against nerves

Pernicious anemia: can be caused by immune system attack of the cells in the lining of your stomach, and causes low B12/poor absorption

Psoriasis: an autoimmune reaction to skin and joints, causing raised, red, scaly patches of skin

Raynaud's (secondary): when blood vessels in fingers and toes over-react to stress or cold, and related to lupus or rheumatoid arthritis

Rheumatoid arthritis: when immune system mistakenly attacks the joints instead of bacteria or viruses

Sjogren's syndrome: attack of glands in eyes and mouth and can progress to other organs

Ulcerative colitis: mixed up immune response towards the lining of the large intestine (colon) and rectum

Vitiligo: when immune system attacks pigment-producing cells in the skin

But don't get too complacent, as there are many more of these autoimmune and autoimmune-related diseases. Here's a full list to knock your socks off by the Autoimmune Registry: *http://www.autoimmuneregistry.org/the-list-1/* If the latter link ever goes bad, just do an internet search for "list of autoimmune diseases".

Here's a potential surprise--below are conditions that might have an autoimmune connection:

- **Fibromyalgia** can have an autoimmune component, since symptoms are so similar to lupus and rheumatoid arthritis.[63] More research is needed.

- **Endometriosis** might have an autoimmune connection since it

---

[63] https://www.ncbi.nlm.nih.gov/pubmed/15082086

shares "elevated levels of cytokines, decreased cell apoptosis, and T- and B-cell abnormalities" with some autoimmune diseases.[64]

- **Lyme disease** may have an autoimmune component. It starts out with the inflammatory effects of the spirochete Borrelia burgdorferi bacteria, but can progress into an autoimmune problem.[65]

The Co-occurrence among many Autoimmune Diseases

Unfortunately, one can find themselves developing other autoimmune conditions with their Hashimoto's — co-occurrences. It's like criminals wanting to hang out with other criminals.

There is even a name for having three autoimmune conditions: Multiple autoimmune syndrome (MAS).

Below are some studies showing connections between two or more, but you'll also see other autoimmune disorder pairings. This is just a sampling.

Please know that these connections don't happen to everyone.
This is more about what autoimmune conditions tend to pair...
if they are going to pair.

- ■ **Hashimoto's in Relation to Other Immune System Disorders and Other Autoimmune Diseases**

One study[66] in the UK found that 14.3% of Hashi's patients also had another autoimmune disease. Additionally, it found that 9.67% of those with Graves' disease had another autoimmune disease. And our own observations of each other as thyroid patients have noticed that for some, the first "other" autoimmune disease may the

[64] https://www.ncbi.nlm.nih.gov/pubmed/11476764
[65] https://www.ncbi.nlm.nih.gov/pubmed/15214872
[66] https://www.ncbi.nlm.nih.gov/pubmed/20103030

pairing of Hashi's with Graves' disease antibodies.

- **Increased Risk of Rheumatoid Arthritis with Hashimoto's**

A study done in Sweden[67] found that the risk was higher that those who were diagnosed with Rheumatoid Arthritis also had had an autoimmune thyroid disease (like Hashimoto's). The question was raised as to which causes what—the chicken or the egg.

- **Hashi's more likely than Graves to have a cluster of Autoimmune diseases**

A European study[68] found that compared to Graves' disease, Hashimoto's was much more likely to cluster with other autoimmune diseases.

- **Increased risk of Down Syndrome with other autoimmune disorders**

Down Syndrome is a genetic disorder caused by the presence of a third copy of chromosome 21. There are characteristic features in the eyes, plus some form of intellectual disability, Observations and research[69] have shown that those with Down Syndrome have an increased risk of having other autoimmune disorders, including Addison's disease, Celiac, diabetes, Graves, Hashimoto's, MS, pernicious anemia, rheumatoid arthritis, Sjogren's syndrome, and lupus.

- **Diabetes type 1 followed by Celiac**

WebMD[70] mentions how both Celiac and Diabetes type 1 autoimmune disorders can go hand-in-hand.

---

[67] https://www.ncbi.nlm.nih.gov/pubmed/30646250
[68] https://www.ncbi.nlm.nih.gov/pubmed/21378091
[69] https://library.down-syndrome.org/en-us/research-practice/12/2/autoimmunity-puz-zle-down-syndrome/
[70] https://www.webmd.com/diabetes/news/20171010/celiac-disease-may-follow-type-1-dia-betes-#1

■ **Hashimoto's with type 1 diabetes mellitus, autoimmune liver diseases and inflammatory bowel disease.**

Some research shows an increased prevalence that one can have these other autoimmune conditions with Hashimoto's.[71]

■ **Hashimoto's with Rheumatoid Arthritis**

Different studies show a connection between the two.[72] [73]

How Hashimoto's can pair with other autoimmune related thyroid problems

Yes. First are two of the most common thyroid related antibodies:

1. **Peroxidase antibody (TPOab):** These are antibodies which attack your peroxidase, which is an enzyme important in the production of thyroid hormones and conversion.
2. **Thyroglobulin antibody (TgAb):** Thyroglobulin are proteins in your thyroid from which thyroid hormones are made.

Sometimes the latter two common thyroid antibodies can pair with antibodies more related to Graves' disease, the hyperthyroid disease:

3. **TSH receptor antibodies (TRAb)** These antibodies are specific to Graves' disease, and stand for TSH receptor antibodies. They usually include **thyroid-stimulating immunoglobulin (TSI) and thyroid blocking antibodies (TBAb)**
4. Other antibodies: **TSH-binding Inhibitor Immunoglobulin (TBII). Thyroid stimulating antibody (TSab). Thyroid-stimulating hormone receptor (TSHR)**

What a mess, don't you think?

---

[71] https://www.ncbi.nlm.nih.gov/pmc/articles/PMC2111403/
[72] https://www.ncbi.nlm.nih.gov/pmc/articles/PMC3505628/
[73] http://www.ejode.eg.net/article.asp?issn=2356-8062;year=2018;volume=4;is-sue=1;spage=5;epage=10;aulast=Abd-Elhafeez

Why do some patients have more than one autoimmune disease?

The answer is unclear, say experts. It's as if one autoimmune disease creates the "path" towards another in some patients. It's also proposed that genetic factors shared between different autoimmune diseases causes the pairing in some individuals.[74]

All in all, it appears that there's a necessity to live as clean as possible, moderate stress, treat gut issues (which we will go over), keep your immune system supported, and avoid known triggers.

TIDBITS

■

- Did you know that the high cortisol from non-autoimmune Cushing's Disease (King Henry VIII of England had this) can protect individuals from autoimmune diseases? Equally, as it's treated and cortisol comes down, the risk of autoimmune diseases goes up in certain individuals.[75]

---

[74] https://www.healio.com/rheumatology/rheumatoid-arthritis/news/print/healio-rheumatolo-gy/%7Bed6a292b-402b-402b-82ca-c2c2e9c01e3b%7D/staying-ahead-of-multiple-autoim-mune-disorders?page=3
[75] https://www.hindawi.com/journals/ije/2018/1464967/

NOTES

Chapter 8

Inflammation

Guess what is a common and highly problematic result of having most autoimmune diseases?

Chronic, expanding, disagreeable inflammation.

In normal and healthy immune responses to pathogens, inflammation is the first tactic and has an important role. For example, when one gets a large and nasty splinter in their finger, that part of the finger will usually become inflamed. Why? It's your body's defense mechanism to protect you from bacteria, viruses, or any other harmful pathogens. That defense mechanism will release certain tiny proteins (cytokines and chemokines) to start the process of inflammatory protection.

Healthy inflammation does the following:
- pinpoints where the injury is
- increases blood flow to the area of injury, allowing more help to flow to the injured area
- seeks to eliminate what is causing the problem
- works to remove any damaged tissue to help healing

But in abnormal autoimmune diseases, inflammation is not just the result of a tissue or gland injury, but the result of an immune system gone haywire---antibodies attacking what they shouldn't be attacking like your tissue or glands.

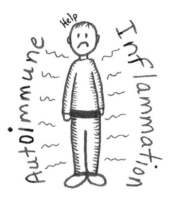

Autoimmune inflammation is the result of the overproduction of those tiny proteins called cytokines and chemokines which are released from the immune system.

Here's a less complicated explanation of what is released from the immune system related to inflammation:

Cytokines refer to a broad category of chemical messenger proteins released by the immune system. They can be pro-inflammatory or anti-inflammatory, and can affect the actions of other cells. Those pro-inflammatory cytokines are involved in chronic pain, for example. They promote either acute or chronic inflammation.

Chemokines are actually smaller versions of the above Cytokines. They are pro-inflammatory. In non-autoimmune situations, they guide cells in the immune system to the site of infection, like little taxis.

The autoimmune overreaction release of these two inflammation proteins is basically an auto-aggressive response by your immune system. It's over-reactive and ends up targeting your tissues and organs.[76]

[76] https://www.researchgate.net/publication/10876044_Cytokines_and_Chemokines_in_Auto-immune_Disease_An_Overview

You might say the autoimmune disease response is just plain overkill. It's like using ten people and their 20 hands to slap an irritating bad guy mosquito on your arm…but in the autoimmune situation, there's no mosquito on the arm being slapped!

And with autoimmune-disease-caused inflammation, it has the potential to go on…and on…and on…like the pink mechanical bunny with sunglasses playing the drum, aka chronic inflammation.

Why is Chronic Inflammation a Concern if Left Unchecked?

The longer inflammation goes, the more damage can be done.

Here are harmful effects of chronic inflammation:

1. A dampening of the feedback loop messaging from the pituitary to the adrenals, meaning your adrenals could start to make less cortisol
2. Rising blood pressure
3. Allergic reactions
4. Uncomfortable and embarrassing swelling
5. Bone loss
6. Uncomfortable joint pain
7. Heart stress
8. High ferritin, your storage iron, causing serum iron to fall
9. Rising reverse T3 (RT3), the inactive hormone causing free T3 to fall and thus resulting in hypothyroid symptoms
10. Other autoimmune inflammation
11. A spread to other tissue and organs

12. Cancer promotion[77]
13. Asthma
14. Sores or rashes
15. Tissue death
16. Other infections or diseases
17. Brain damage or dementia
18. Buildup of plaque
19. Internal scarring
20. Weight gain
21. Insomnia
22. Depression
23. Anxiety from high cortisol
24. Constipation or diarrhea
25. Acid reflux

Lab Work Needed to Detect Inflammation

Three examples of lab work to detect inflammation.[78]

Ferritin (iron storage) This will rise in the presence of inflammation, i.e. the body will throw any iron from food or supplements into storage to protect you from feeding inflammation. So, for women, that would be a ferritin close to 100 or above, or for men, in the 120s or above—the latter based on years of observations and reports by patients with inflammation. Ferritin ranges are ridiculously broad in most cases, i.e. 12 to 150 ng/mL for women, and 12 to 300 for men. If your lab facility's range is different, you can analyze where the results mentioned above fall in those ranges, and make a similar analysis of your provided range.

---

[77] https://www.ncbi.nlm.nih.gov/pmc/articles/PMC2803035/
[78] http://stopthethyroidmadness.com/inflammation

CRP (C-Reactive Protein) This is a substance produced by the liver in response to inflammation.

ESR (erythrocyte sedimentation rate) This measures how fast your red blood cells fall to the bottom of the tube, indicating inflammation.

Why Three Labs to Detect Inflammation?

Three labs can sometimes be needed because inflammation can be expressed differently between individuals[79]. Granted, it appears that most will have high ferritin reflecting inflammation, since inflammation will push iron into storage, thus testing ferritin. But some have low or good ferritin and too-high CRP or ESR.

What is an Action Plan for Autoimmune-Caused Inflammation?

The action plan includes what patients have reported in the treatment of Hashimoto's, as you will see compiled in Chapter 16.

- lowering antibodies
- using the right thyroid medication like natural desiccated thyroid (NDT), synthetic T4/T3, or T3-only and being **optimal,** not just "on them". See *http://stopthethyroidmadness.com/lab-values*
- treating non-optimal or low iron levels
- treating a cortisol problem
- using specific supplements to counter and lower inflammation[80]
- avoiding inflammation triggering foods (See Chapter 13)
- moderating life's stresses—very important

[79] http://stopthethyroidmadness.com/inflammation
[80] http://stopthethyroidmadness.com/inflammation

- identifying and treating bacterial or viral infections
- avoiding mold exposure
- treating candida overgrowth
- keeping nutrient levels optimal.
- understanding and eliminating food triggers

Inflammation Lowering Supplements

READ ME: it's important to be responsible and investigate any supplement listed below to make sure you have no sensitivity to any of these, plus potential side effects. I also like using supplement sites with legitimate reviews as part my own discernment as to what is good to take. Many patients state taking more than one, but it's never about taking" massive" amounts of a combination of any of the below. That can stress the liver!

- **Selenium[81]:** (patients often test first though, to make sure it's not too high already due to a methylation problem like MTHFR, etc) Selenium is involved in regulating the overreactive, inflammation-causing immune responses in Hashi's. 200 to 400 mcg max is the oft-mentioned safe amount.

- **Astaxanthin[82]:** Antioxidant found in pink-tinted ocean organisms like lobster, shrimp, salmon, etc. Known to reduce inflammation. 12 mg is a commonly used amount.

- **Bioflavanoids[83]:** can be found in citrus fruits, green tea, berries, onions and even red wine.

---

[81] https://www.ncbi.nlm.nih.gov/pmc/articles/PMC3277928/
[82] https://nutritionandmetabolism.biomedcentral.com/articles/10.1186/1743-7075-7-18
[83] https://www.hindawi.com/journals/jir/2018/9324357/

- **Serrapeptase**[84]**:** an enzyme from silkworms known to be anti-inflammatory. 120,000 units it commonly mentioned. It can thin blood, so watch for that.

- **Glucosamine and chondroitin**[85]**:** powerful anti-inflammatory in combination.

- **Pau D'Arco tea**[86]**:** from the bark of a tree and known to help lower inflammation.

- **Ginger**[87]**:** a top nutrient, as it's anti-inflammatory, besides providing pain relief due to the inflammation. When I used to be on Synthroid, I took ginger in caps for inflammation pain in my fingers called tendonitis—the latter caused by the inadequate treatment of Synthroid. After a week or so, the inflammation went down!

- **Curcumin**[88]**:** Curcumin is the anti-inflammatory substance found in the spice called turmeric. Some take higher amounts than the bottle says if countering inflammation, such as 5 in the morning; 5 in the evening, then less. WARNING: some people have an allergy to curcumin, so you might want to test first. Side effects in a minority are headache and nausea.

- **Cinnamon**[89]**:** another spice with inflammatory properties. Can be stirred or mixed into a favorite, tolerable food. There are even cinnamon capsules! Don't take too much--thins blood.

- **Rosehips**[90]**:** anti-inflammatory and specifically for certain autoimmune inflammation[91]

- **Guggul**[92]**:** Ayurveda treatment/plant based; said to be equal to the effects of aspirin or ibuprofen. 500 mg three times a day.

---

84 https://www.lifeextension.com/magazine/2003/9/report_aas/Page-01
85 https://www.ncbi.nlm.nih.gov/pmc/articles/PMC4048982/
86 https://selfhacked.com/blog/pau-darco-tree/
87 https://www.ncbi.nlm.nih.gov/pmc/articles/PMC3665023/
88 https://www.sciencedirect.com/science/article/pii/S0278691515001878
89 https://www.healthline.com/nutrition/10-proven-benefits-of-cinnamon
90 https://www.ncbi.nlm.nih.gov/pubmed/22762068
91 https://www.ncbi.nlm.nih.gov/pubmed/22762068
92 https://www.ncbi.nlm.nih.gov/pubmed/18078436

- **Cat's Claw**[93]: treats inflammation (by suppressing TNF-alpha synthesis–which is needed in the inflammation process)
- **Boswellia (Frankincense)**[94]: Herbal extract which is known to help lower inflammatory response.
- **Fish oil**[95]: Stated to reduce the inflammatory response with its omega 3 content
- **Holy Basil/Tulsi**[96]: anti-inflammatory member of mint family and sweet basil, high vitamin K content, anti-histamine and it can help with high blood sugar issues. Patients also use it to lower high cortisol. It's not a long-term treatment.
- **Chlorella**[97]: freshwater algae that has anti-inflammatory benefits
- **Berberine**[98]: can help lower blood sugars and clear inflammation
- **Neem**[99]: from the neem tree and anti-inflammatory
- **Bromelain**[100]: found in pineapple and has inflammation-lowering properties
- **Cilantro**[101]: ayurvedic medicinal herb that is known to lower inflammation. Some suggest taking it in smaller amounts and with a binding agent, such as chlorella. Tastes good except to those with certain genetics that causes it to taste bad.
- **Slippery Elm**[102]: anti-inflammatory and stated especially for GI complaints. Can coat the stomach, which may be desired.
- **Pink Rock Rose (Cistus Incanus)**[103]: has anti-inflammatory, antioxidant, antibacterial, and anti-viral properties

---

[93] http://heartofwellness.org/the-anti-inflammatory-power-of-cats-claw/
[94] https://selfhacked.com/blog/boswellia/
[95] https://www.ncbi.nlm.nih.gov/pubmed/16531187
[96] https://www.hindawi.com/journals/ecam/2017/9217567/
[97] https://www.healthline.com/nutrition/benefits-of-chlorella
[98] https://www.ncbi.nlm.nih.gov/pmc/articles/PMC3942282/
[99] https://www.ncbi.nlm.nih.gov/pmc/articles/PMC4791507/
[100] https://www.ncbi.nlm.nih.gov/pmc/articles/PMC3529416/
[101] https://draxe.com/cilantro-benefits/
[102] https://selfhacked.com/blog/slippery-elm/
[103] https://mindbodyyes.com/cistus-incanus-health-benefits/

■ **Resveratrol**[104]: component of red wine and grapes, especially the skin of the grapes, with evidence of anti-inflammatory effects; start low and build to prevent side-effects.

Anti-Inflammatory Foods

Just as there are inflammation-promoting foods to consider and avoid (Chapter 13), it turns out that certain other foods are anti-inflammatory! Here are examples of anti-inflammatory foods to explore and have in your diet:

- Avocados [105]
- Berries [106]
- Broccoli, cabbage and brussel sprouts in moderation [107]
- Chia seeds [108]
- Dark leafy greens
- Fatty fish like salmon with its omega 3[109]
- Fiber-rich foods
- Fresh ginger [110]
- Grapes [111]
- Green and black tea [112]
- Pomegranates [113]
- Tart Cherries [114]

---

[104] https://medicalxpress.com/news/2016-09-resveratrol-inflammation.html
[105] https://www.ncbi.nlm.nih.gov/pmc/articles/PMC3664913/
[106] https://www.ncbi.nlm.nih.gov/pubmed/26501271
[107] https://www.ncbi.nlm.nih.gov/pubmed/21129940
[108] https://www.researchgate.net/publication/322934474_Chia_protein_concentrate_Salvia_hispanica_l_anti-inflammatory_and_antioxidant_activity
[109] https://www.healthline.com/nutrition/11-benefits-of-salmon
[110] https://www.ncbi.nlm.nih.gov/pmc/articles/PMC3665023/
[111] https://www.ncbi.nlm.nih.gov/pmc/articles/PMC3546615/
[112] https://www.ncbi.nlm.nih.gov/pmc/articles/PMC3401676/
[113] https://www.ncbi.nlm.nih.gov/pubmed/23573120
[114] https://www.ncbi.nlm.nih.gov/pmc/articles/PMC5872786/

Anti-Inflammatory Diets

1. Autoimmune Paleo Diet (AIP)[115]

If you prefer to use a diet specifically geared towards being anti-inflammatory, AIP is it. Be prepared that it's a very strict diet. But it can be worth it to finally control chronic inflammation. Many patients move from AIP to the Paleo diet after the AIP has done its job.

There are numerous websites which explain it, and here's a great one, too: https://aiplifestyle.com/what-is-autoimmune-protocol-diet/ And this one: *https://unboundwellness.com/*

There are also numerous books/cookbooks to help, as well, including The Autoimmune Paleo Cookbook: An Allergen-Free Approach to Managing Chronic Illness by Mickey Trescott

AIP acceptable foods

- meats
- fish
- various veggies
- fruits
- sweet potatoes
- coconut milk
- oils like avocado, coconut, olive
- vinegar
- bone broth
- fermented foods without dairy
- honey in moderation
- non-seed herbs and teas

---

[115] https://www.ncbi.nlm.nih.gov/pmc/articles/PMC5647120/

Foods to avoid on AIP diet

- all grains
- all dairy
- all sugar
- eggs
- beans
- peanuts
- tomatoes
- eggplant
- peppers
- potatoes
- butter and ghee
- all oils except those listed above
- food additives
- alcohol

2. Paleo diet

This diet is less strict than the AIP with a focus on foods that our hunter-gatherer ancestors may have consumed, i.e. whole, unprocessed, anti-inflammatory foods.

Examples of acceptable Paleo diet foods:

- grass-fed meats
- fish, wild caught
- chicken
- bacon
- fruits
- veggies
- eggs
- nuts
- seeds
- oils like avocado, coconut, olive and more

Like AIP, there are numerous Paleo books and cookbooks, like *"The Paleo Thyroid Solution: Stop Feeling Fat, Foggy, And Fatigued At The Hands Of Uninformed Doctors - Reclaim Your Health!"* by Elle Russ. Check them out!

TIDBITS

- Studies[116] can show that just 20 minutes of brisk walking can help against inflammation.

- Good news for all chocolate lovers---dark chocolate in moderation is anti-inflammatory[117]!

---

[116] https://www.sciencedirect.com/science/article/pii/S0889159116305645
[117] https://www.scientificamerican.com/article/why-is-dark-chocolate-good-for-you-thank-your-microbes/

NOTES

Chapter 9

Your Gut
Part 1:
the Hashimoto's
Smoking Gun

L et's now explore a prominent, trigger-pulling "bam!" for the onset-or-worsening of Hashimoto's disease: **having a compromised or problematic gut.**

In other words, just as genetics can play a strong underlying role for developing autoimmune diseases like Hashimoto's, **problems in your gastrointestinal tract** are most likely an enormous provoking factor towards that Hashi's, as well.

And why are problems in your gut an itchy finger towards Hashimoto's disease? *Because your GI tract is where up to 80% of your immune function does its job...but in autoimmune- susceptible individuals, that can mean the attack on your thyroid, too.*

Your digestive system is where...
- barriers are in place against any pathogens
- inflammation can be set off against those bad guys,
- a diverse population of gut bacteria promote better immune function
- immune cells can excrete antibodies to deal with bad guys

So, if something goes wrong with the beneficial bacteria or mucus barriers, or if an invading bad guy sneaked into your gut and causes a rise in your antibodies to fight it, imagine what all that can mean in triggering or fanning the flames of Hashimoto's in susceptible individuals…[118]

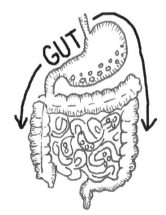

Immune System and the Gut

To put us on the same page, "gut" refers to your gastrointestinal tract, aka the "GI tract". It's a series of open, hollow organs which constitutes the journey from your mouth (that which goes into the body like food and water) to your anus (where what is not used/ broken down goes out).

What comes out? It's the remains of food not absorbed and broken down by your gut bacteria.[119] It also contains some of your gut bacteria, metabolic waste products like bilirubin, and dead cells which once lined the gut.

And of course, the gut is also about what occurs in-between: in the esophagus, stomach, and the small and large intestines. Additionally, the GI tract function involves solid organs as well: your liver (the filter plus producer of bile), gallbladder (the storage of bile and the releaser) and pancreas (produces insulin and digestive enzymes).[120]

In a simple explanation, your GI Tract is an
interior bodily system which…

---

[118] https://www.ncbi.nlm.nih.gov/pubmed/23200063
[119] https://en.wikipedia.org/wiki/Human_feces
[120] https://www.niddk.nih.gov/health-information/digestive-diseases/digestive-sys-tem-how-it-works

- takes in the food you eat
- digests that food to absorb important nutrients
- expels as feces

Your gut is also working to maintain the right balance between the entrance of what is good (nutrient rich foods) vs countering the entrance of what is bad (pathogens).

Mostly though, the reference to your "gut" in this chapter is going to pertain to your stomach and intestines. But there will be mention of solid organs as well.

And here's where a normal, healthy body is wise.

When it's healthy, balanced, and doing its job like a well-oiled machine, one's GI tract has important functions that act as your immune system to protect and defend you against harmful toxins that might come in via food or what your mouth or saliva alone brings in, i.e. viruses, bad bacteria, parasites and more.

For example …

- **Mucosal barrier:** This is a layer of mucus, secreted by epithelial cells, which lines your stomach and even your intestines. It not only lubricates your food for easier movement, but as part of the immune system, it helps keep the acid in your stomach as a first line of defense against certain food-carried, saliva-carried pathogens. This mucosal layer also allows nutrients to come into your body while protecting you against toxins, i.e. it's antimicrobial.

- **Gut Flora:** This term primarily describes the many different strains of bacteria that populate your intestines. And within the bacteria mix should be a heavy percentage and variety of good and beneficial bacteria—all with many roles to help maintain your immune health! These good bacteria end up teaching your immune system that not everything down there is bad.

■ **Gut-associated lymphoid tissue (GALT):** This is a component
of the mucus layer which stores immune cells like T and B
lymphocytes, ready to strike against pathogens like mighty
knights in armor. The T cells recognize antigens (bad guys)
outside infected cells, and the B cells recognize the bad guys
on the surface of bacteria and viruses.[121] It's the B cells that
produce and release antibodies, activating the immune system
to destroy the pathogens.

**But what happens if my gut is not healthy, balanced,
and doing its job well?**

The simple answer is that a gut with problems raises your risk
to develop an autoimmune problem like Hashimoto's, and most
especially for those with an inherited genetic propensity. Or a
problematic gut exacerbates Hashi's that is already active—it's like
pouring salt on a wound. Ouch.

In turn, developing or worsening Hashimoto's disease increases
your risk of hypothyroidism because of the attack. Being hypothyroid
causes all sorts of problems, ranging from fatigue, easy weight gain,
dry skin and hair, hair loss, depression, anxiety, cortisol problems,
low iron, low B12, low other nutrients...on and on.

Issues to discover: Strategies to Improve Gut Health

Check out these 10 potential gut issues that you'll want to discover and
treat, both in this chapter and the next. They are in no particular order as
all can be very problematic! Eight are in this chapter, and the final two are
in Chapter 10.

---

[121] https://www.researchgate.net/publication/320182585_Difference_Between_T_Cells_and_B_Cells

HASHIMOTO'S GUT PROBLEM #1:
Poor Levels of Digestive Enzymes

The pancreas, which sits behind your stomach, makes important digestive enzymes. They help you break down / digest your food, especially those fats, proteins and carbs, in order to create smaller absorbable nutrients for your health and well-being. It's all important for a strong gut function. Those enzymes include:

- **Amylase:** converts glycogen and starch (carbohydrates) into simple sugars. Those simple sugars then make their way through you blood to your cells, providing energy. They can also be stored for future use.
- **Protease:** helps break down and digest the peptide bond / amino acids in proteins. You need proteins to make other enzymes and to be used for bones, cartilage, muscles, and skin.
- **Lipase:** helps breaks down fats. Fats are needed for energy and cell growth. Fats are needed for your mitochondria. They are a great backup if you aren't breaking down carbs well.

And for various reasons, one's levels of digestive enzymes can drop, or the body fails to use them correctly.

Causes of Lowered Enzymes
- getting older
- high heavy metals, plus the detox stressing one's pancreas
- low stomach acid symptoms (acid reflux, poor nutrient levels)
- gallstones (could cause pain)
- stomach ulcers
- genetic mutations[122]

---

[122] https://www.hindawi.com/journals/scientica/2016/9828672/

- alcohol abuse
- chronically eating until full, which can deplete your enzymes

Any of these autoimmune diseases can lower your enzymes
- Lupus: autoimmune disease against tissues
- Crohn's: autoimmune disease of the bowels
- Celiac disease: autoimmune reaction against gluten
- Pancreatitis: inflammation of the pancreas
- Cystic fibrosis: genetic disorder mostly affecting the lungs
- Shwachman-Diamond syndrome: condition causing pancreatic insufficiency plus bone marrow dysfunction

Symptoms of Low Enzymes

Check out this list of symptoms of an inadequate release of pancreative digestive enzymes:

- may be silent
- low nutrient levels via testing—a biggie
- crashing easily with fatigue
- excess gas or bloating
- can promote SIBO (small intestinal bacterial overgrowth)
- diarrhea
- cramping
- seeing undigested food in stools
- bad smelling stools or those that float (can also be caused by low bile due to a gallbladder issue)
- cravings for certain foods
- feeling tired after eating
- breakouts on face like acne
- the need to eat often to prevent grouchiness
- risk of Hashimoto's

Testing for Low Enzymes

Since symptoms of low enzymes might be similar to symptoms of other problems, testing can be ideal.

- Organic Acids Test (OAT) by Great Plains which you order yourself. It can show levels not being broken down.
- Samples of saliva, blood or stool to test for digestive enzymatic presence or absence by your doctor. This is an ideal way to find out.

Treatment for Low Enzymes

- foods with natural digestive enzymes like kefir, sauerkraut, honey, ginger, kiwi fruit, papaya, pineapple, mango, bananas, avocados,
- consuming bitters before meals to help promote digestive enzymes—bitters are a mixture of some alcohol with certain herbs, roots, fruit, bark, leaves, etc.
- supplemental enzymes like Dr. Amy Myers version called Complete Enzymes, or for more serious pancreas sluggishness, Pure Encapsulations Pancreatic Enzyme formula
- Research[123] shows that coconut oil stimulates the lipase digestive enzyme.
- The pancreas need zinc, magnesium, manganese and other minerals to perform at its best.

HASHIMOTO'S GUT PROBLEM #2:
Low Stomach Acid

Stomach/gastric acid in the right amounts is critical. It helps break down foods and proteins properly, helps absorb nutrients, helps B12

---

[123] https://www.ncbi.nlm.nih.gov/pubmed/10827346

absorption, keeps food from sitting in the stomach too long, protects against bacteria and bacterial overgrowth, stimulates the release of bile, helps open and close the pyloric sphincter at the top of your stomach.

Causes of Low Stomach Acid

- being on T4-only medications like Synthroid, generic levothyroxine, Eltroxin, Oroxine, etc.
- being underdosed on natural desiccated thyroid, T4/T3 or T3-only, usually by doctors who hold you hostage to the TSH[124], or are simply afraid to raise.
- zinc deficiency
- b-vitamin deficiency
- chronic stress
- aging (darn it!)
- smoking
- alcohol excess
- chronic inflammation
- certain food sensitivities
- antibiotic overuse
- anything that messes with our stomach bacteria
- excess sugar consumption as well as processed foods
- overuse of NSAIDS, aka aspirin, acetaminophen, or ibuprofen

Symptoms of Low Stomach Acid

- acid reflux (yes, most of the time, that's due to LOW stomach acid, not high). See *http://stopthethyroidmadness.com/stomach-acid*
- risk of Hashimoto's from poor nutrient absorption

---

[124] http://stopthethyroidmadness.com.tsh-why-its-useless

- gut inflammation
- leaky gut
- poor digestion; food sitting in stomach
- low nutrient absorption
- bloating
- cramps
- gas, and especially foul smelling
- undigested food in stools

Treatment of Low Stomach Acid

- Betaine HCL supplementation with food. Some also contain the beneficial peptides

- Up to a tablespoon of lemon juice or apple cider vinegar mixed with water (can be flavored of your choice). They are natural acids, and may even stimulate your own production over time.

- Eat those pickles, fermented cabbage, kefir drink, kombucha tea, sauerkraut —they naturally improve stomach acid levels

- Same as above but with lemon juice and sweetener like stevia, if needed.

- Lower inflammation with curcumin, ginger, bromelain.

> **WARNING!** Be careful if your doctor suggests an acid-blocking supplement or med! Most Hashi's patients do NOT have too much stomach acid causing problems. They have too little due to their hypothyroidism. If in doubt, test.

HASHIMOTO'S GUT PROBLEM #3:
Consuming Inflammation-Promoting Foods

Hashimoto's is always about inflammation.

Thus, foods which can promote inflammation can not only tip the scales towards Hashimoto's, but can also promote more inflammation on top of the inflammation Hashi's already causes due to the autoimmune attack. Then, there comes the inflammation just from being hypothyroid due to T4-only medications[125]. It's a vicious inflammation circle!

For those susceptible to certain foods (and many with Hashi's are very vulnerable), it's helpful to avoid or lower the consumption of these foods which might promote further inflammation, rising antibodies, and worsening symptoms. *We've seen repeatedly that it can be individual as to which of the below will cause inflammation in susceptible individuals.*

Problematic foods can include (but are not limited to):
- most grains
- dairy
- nightshades
- sugar or anything that spikes your insulin
- eggs
- gluten-containing foods
- corn

Remember that it's individual what foods cause reactions in those who carry a risk of autoimmune problems, or for those who already

---

[125] http://stopthethyroidmadness.com/t4-only-meds-dont-work

have Hashimoto's disease. But the latter as a whole is a common group of foods stated to promote inflammation.

Instead, focusing on nutrient rich foods gives your gut a better, less inflammatory environment.[126]

Nutrient rich, anti-inflammatory foods include:

- Vegetables with color like kale, dark leafy greens and asparagus, plus carrots, celery, green or red peppers (only if you tolerate them) and more. (I'm not a big veggie eater, so I tend to put them in a blender with frozen berries to create a cold thick drink)

- Blueberries are rich in anti-inflammatory antioxidants. Same with Montmorency tart cherries. Also consider strawberries and other berries.

- Good fats like MCT oil, coconut oil, flaxseed oil (rather than canola or corn oils).

- Avocados

- Macadamia nuts are high in antioxidants and fiber, which can help reduce inflammation.

- Beets (or beet root juice) are high in antioxidants and can help reduce inflammation.

- Tomatoes (only if you tolerate them) are rich in lycopene's which help reduce inflammation

- Grass fed beef

- Fish like salmon (though not farmed salmon—too many potential toxins), sardines and shellfish if you tolerate them

- Kefir and kombucha fermented drinks if you tolerate them.

---

[126] https://www.consciouslifestylemag.com/nutrient-dense-foods/

HASHIMOTO'S GUT PROBLEM #4:
Gluten

Gluten is a particularly bad problem for the vast majority of Hashimoto's patients! No kidding and no exaggeration.

There are five kinds of gluten problems[127]. The first three are autoimmune related:

1. **Celiac disease (CD)** - This can be a common autoimmune disease with Hashimoto's since autoimmune problems can pair up, sooner or later.

2. **Gluten ataxia**[128] - This a rarer autoimmune condition where the antibodies released in response to gluten attack the brain.

3. **Dermatitis herpetiformis (DH)**[129] - This is an itchy skin manifestation due to gluten that can also cause skin blisters and be very chronic. There are IgA antibodies, and this is usually associated with Celiac.

Then two more are not autoimmune related:

4. **Non-celiac gluten sensitivity (NCGS)** - I had a good friend with this and it was pretty severe, driving her inflammation quite high.

5. **Wheat allergy** - IgE-mediated and non-IgE-mediated. Symptoms are often immediate after consuming wheat, or within two hours.

Even Dr. Tom O'Bryan, DC, CCN, DACBN [130], a global expert about gluten,

---

[127] https://en.wikipedia.org/wiki/Gluten-related_disorders
[128] https://www.ncbi.nlm.nih.gov/pubmed/18787912
[129] https://www.ncbi.nlm.nih.gov/pubmed/8256113
[130] https://thedr.com/

underscores that there can be over 300 autoimmune diseases related to gluten. You can view his website here: *https://thedr.com/*

Gluten refers to glue-like proteins, gliadin and glutenin, which when mixed with water, combine and hold certain bread products together. It also traps those gas bubbles in the dough rising process (thus the empty oval and round spaces you see in bread), and gives that chewy texture you notice when biting into bread.

Those gluten-forming proteins are found in grains like *barley, bulgur, oats, rye and different forms of wheat*. But gluten can be in so many other foods! The Celiac Disease Foundation has a great list of gluten grains as well as gluten-containing foods, whether you just have gluten intolerance making Hashi's worse, or Celiac. *https://celiac. org/gluten-free-living/what-is-gluten/sources-of-gluten/* Or you can just do an internet search for "foods containing gluten".

For the majority of Hashimoto's patients, consuming gluten-containing foods is a big problem.

Why? Because the protein structure of gluten will too closely resemble your thyroid tissue—that which your overreactive antibodies want to attack. Thus, you can see a rise of your autoimmune antibodies as well as inflammation.

Gluten consumption can also cause symptoms, depending on the individual, like headaches, fatigue, skin issues, depression, diarrhea, smelly stools, bloating and more. Chapter 13 contains reported symptoms from gluten, and there are a lot!

Granted, there is a very small minority who report no issue with gluten...yet. But since the majority do, it's definitely a problem to be aware of, aka *any form of gluten intolerance*.

Then there are those who have the serious and inherited autoimmune issue caused Celiac Disease. It's a disorder in which gluten can cause a damaged intestinal mucosa. The attack in the small intestine can lead to damage of the tiny projections that line the intestine, called villi. Thus, absorption of nutrients is severely compromised.

The bottom line is that most reading this, who have an autoimmune tendency, should be committed to removing all sources of gluten from one's diet. It's just not worth the problems it causes. When you get to Chapter 13, you'll see all the problems patients report from consuming gluten—it's not a pretty picture.

HASHIMOTO'S GUT PROBLEM #5:
The Wrong Thyroid Medications

Why is treating your hypothyroid state related to the gut? Because the wrong medications negatively affect the gut, as we've seen for years now in patients and their reports.

In the updated revised book *"Stop the Thyroid Madness: A Patient Revolution Against Decades of Inferior Thyroid Treatment",* I explain how the introduction of T4-only medications around 1960 has been a huge scandal in the treatment of hypothyroidism, whether caused by Hashimoto's or not. Why? Because T4, a thyroid storage hormone, is only one of five well-known thyroid hormones. Its purpose is to convert to the active hormone T3.

Yet… a healthy thyroid also gives you some direct T3, the active hormone!! It's not forcing you to get all your T3 from conversion.

> Forcing the body to live for conversion alone on T4-only has been a disaster for millions worldwide all these decades. Sooner or later, patients report seeing clear symptoms of continued hypothyroidism on T4-only, aka Synthroid, Levothyroxine, Eltroxin, Oroxine, or a number of other T4-only brands.

The symptoms of continued hypothyroidism while on T4-only include, but are not limited to...

- inflammation
- easy fatigue
- poor stamina
- depression
- the need for naps
- hair loss
- dry skin
- dry hair
- hair loss
- anxiety
- weight gain
- difficulty losing
- rising or high cholesterol
- rising or high blood pressure
- fibromyalgia symptoms
- an overreactive autonomic nervous system (I had this)
- joint pain
- stiffness
- getting sicker than others from illnesses
- bottom of feet pain
- cortisol problems like adrenal fatigue or high cortisol
- falling stomach acid
- low iron
- low B12
- low vitamin D
- low other nutrients

I could go on and on and on as to what patients have reported happened to them on T4-only, sooner or later. Check out the solid information in Chapter 1 in the updated revision of the book *Stop the Thyroid Madness: A Patient Revolution Against Decades of Inferior Treatment*

Why is Treating with just Thyroxine / T4 a Problem for One's Gut?

Treating with simply a thyroid storage hormone (T4) ends up leaving millions with continued hypothyroidism in their own degree and kind, sooner or later. And with all the problems it causes, that also means your metabolism is slower than it should be.

What a slow metabolism due to T4 meds can do to you as a Hashimoto's patient:

- Lower your stomach acid, which lowers nutrient absorption
- Raise the risk of h-pylori, a bad bacteria in your gut
- Cause acid reflux
- Slow the digestion and absorption of food
- Lower important nutrient levels

Besides the following...

- Stresses your immune function
- Keeps you feeling less than optimal
- Raises the risk of heart and bone problems
- Stresses your adrenals leading to high cortisol, then low cortisol

So now, in addition to the challenges you face with an autoimmune condition like Hashimoto's, and whatever other autoimmune condition your Hashi's is paired with, you now have more issues to push you down, down, down.

What works better than T4-only medications?

In order of efficacy according to the reports and experiences of hypothyroid patients worldwide...

1. Natural Desiccated Thyroid (NDT) with optimal levels
2. Synthetic T4 with Synthetic T3 with optimal levels
3. T3-only with optimal levels

And even on these better medications, it's important to be optimal in the ranges, not just "in range". And to get there, we found out the hard way over the years that we have to have optimal iron and cortisol! If you don't, problems happen when raising.

> Optimal for most on NDT or T4/T3 seems to put the free T3 toward the top part of the provided range, and the free T4 around mid-range. Both. On T3 alone, optimal seems to be at the very top if not slightly over, say patients over the years.

But...to get there without reactions or problems (which causes people to wrongly blame the medication), it's important that iron and cortisol be optimal, too, to avoid problems raising these meds, like hyper-like symptoms of anxiety, heart palps, fast heart rate, etc. The website and page explain the importance of iron and cortisol:

http://stopthethyroidmadness.com/iron-and-cortisol

At this point, I want to challenge you to read the Stop the Thyroid Madness (STTM) website *http://stopthethyroidmadness.com* and the STTM books, especially the updated revision Stop the Thyroid Madness book. This patient-to-patient book will teach you how patients use NDT successfully (or T4 with T3, or T3-only), how they have learned to read lab work (which has nothing to do with falling in those normal ranges), how they treat other issues, and more.

HASHIMOTO'S GUT PROBLEM #6:
High Heavy Metals

Yes, having high heavy metals in your body can negatively affect your gut.[131]

---

[131] https://www.ncbi.nlm.nih.gov/pmc/articles/PMC3874687/

I once found myself with high copper and lead. And I personally found that the detox of those metals must have horrifically affected my gut health, as well. Why? Because after the first 6-month detox, I found myself with SIBO. I have never in my life had gut problems...until this happened to me. I also had two miserable experiences with candida from hell.

It turns out that the high heavy metals and the detox had stressed my liver (which produces bile), my gallbladder (which stores bile) and my pancreas (releases digestive enzymes). And insufficient bile is a risk factor for both SIBO and candida! I also dealt with worsening low stomach acid after this incident.

Research also shows that heavy metal exposure can negatively alter your important gut bacteria.[132] [133]

HASHIMOTO'S GUT PROBLEM #7:
Liver or Gallbladder Problems Causing Low Bile Levels

Whether the inadequate levels of bile are coming from either liver stress or blockages, or from problems in the gallbladder, it's a problematic situation for your gut health, since bile serves to remove toxins and break down fats for energy.

Issues that can be caused by inadequate bile:

- Increased intestinal permeability, aka leaky gut (just as the right levels protect the gut lining)[134].
- Increased inflammation (just as the right levels reduce inflammation).[135]

---

[132] https://www.nature.com/articles/s41598-018-24931-w
[133] http://engine.scichina.com/publisher/scp/journal/SB/62/12/10.1016/j.scib.2017.01.031?slug=abstract
[134] https://www.ncbi.nlm.nih.gov/pubmed/18239063
[135] https://www.ncbi.nlm.nih.gov/pubmed/27586800

- Hinderance of the digestive breakdown and absorption of fat (just as the right levels promote better fat breakdown.)[136]
- Inadequate vitamins A, D, E, and K due to poor fat breakdown.[137]
- Increased likelihood of diarrhea and/or erratic bowel movements
- Increase of toxins and waste products in your body—definitely not good for your gut health!
- Particularly smelly gas; ragged-edge stools
- Headache or migraines

Types of Gallbladder Problems:
The Merck Manual[138] lists these:
- Gallstones which block bile ducts
- Injury to bile ducts due to gallbladder surgery
- Narrowing of bile ducts from AIDS
- Pancreatic disorders which narrow bile ducts of pancreases
- Tumors in the pancreas, gallbladder, or bile ducts

Plus, more:
- Gallbladder inflammation called Cholecystitis
- Bile duct stones, aka choledocholithiasis
- Gallbladder cancer (luckily very rare!)
- Bile duct infection
- Gallbladder sludge

Treatment for Low Bile
This is one area where I strongly recommend you find a knowledgeable doctor to help you!

---

[136] http://www.vivo.colostate.edu/hbooks/pathphys/digestion/liver/bile.html
[137] https://www.ncbi.nlm.nih.gov/pmc/articles/PMC2863217/
[138] https://www.merckmanuals.com/home/liver-and-gallbladder-disorders/gallbladder-and-bile-duct-disorders/overview-of-gallbladder-and-bile-duct-disorders

Recommendations for ways to stimulate bile: supplementation with bitters, curcumin, milk thistle, dandelion root and ginger. I have no patient experiences if they work.

Dissolving gallstones is a different story: recommendations are high dose vitamin C[139] plus a drink of apple juice with vinegar every day—the latter to lower the liver's production of cholesterol, of which gallstones are made. Peppermint oil in capsules is another idea. Or a juice made up of beetroots, carrot and cucumbers.

I like what Chris Kressler, founder of the Kressler Institute, says on his website[140]. It's about doing the right tests (ALT, AST, plus bilirubin and more), to remove inflammatory foods, to break the inflammation by healing the gut, stimulate bile flow with certain supplements like Milk Thistle, and take bile salt supplements, if needed. Check out his excellent article and website here for every more details: *https://kresslerinstitute.com*

Until one figures out the cause of low bile, one brand of bile salts is called Cholacol and seems to be an excellent supplement to give yourself back the bile you aren't getting.

My story with a Gallbladder Problem

In 2013, I accidentally inhaled massive amounts of mold spores from the wet dirt I was kicking up while leaf blowing. And no telling what other poisons were in that dirt from years of bug spraying done around the perimeter of the house.

As a result, I was sick as a dog for three miserable months after inhaling what I did—the worst I have ever felt in my life

---

[139] https://onlinelibrary.wiley.com/doi/abs/10.1046/j.1365-2362.1997.1240670.x
[140] https://kresserinstitute.com/little-known-connection-leaky-gut-gluten-intolerance-gallbladder-problems/

along with massive daily fatigue from an immune system in great overdrive. I slowly healed with the help of my doctor, but great damage had been done. It lowered many nutrients like zinc, which caused high copper by 2015. I even found myself with high lead.

When I did my first detox of the high metals in 2015 that lasted 6 months, I was debilitated with fatigue from the detox. I didn't realize it yet, but that fatigue was because my mitochondria were showing evidence of poor functioning. I then found myself with SIBO. Why did that happen, I wondered? I had never had SIBO in my life before that.

Hidden at first was the fact that all that stress with toxins stressed my liver and gallbladder. Testing showed by later 2015 that I wasn't breaking down fats at all. But why? I had no idea, until 2018! A wise doctor suggested my gallbladder. And as symptoms of a gallbladder problem increased in 2018, it was taking bile tablets which saved me.

Once I got on that bile in late 2018 (Cholacol, 1-2 tablets per meal), I saw major improvements in issues that bewildered me. Taking bile improved twenty-one issues that were revealed on an Organic Acid Test (OAT) by Great Plains in early 2019. The most profound improvement was in my mitochondrial function. I had six areas that proved my mito was being dysfunctional, and apparently, taking bile reversed all six of them!!

Why did bile improve so many issues in me? Bile was helping me finally break down fat, as revealed by my OAT test. And fatty acids are needed for your mitochondria! Bile also helps the absorption of vitamins A, D, E, and K. So I additionally started to see chronic issues in my gut start to heal.

HASHIMOTO'S GUT PROBLEM #8:
Parasites

Just one more trigger towards Hashimoto's or making it worse: parasites. A parasite is an organism that feeds on another organism, which in this case could be you. Additionally, while it's gorging on you, it can spread disease.

Parasites can be very tiny, or very long like worms. I recently saw a photo of a parasite that someone pulled out of their rectum...and it was long....ick!!!

Most parasites prefer your intestinal wall as their food home— your gut!

How you acquire parasites

1. Sadly, if you love sushi with that raw or undercooked meat, there is a risk you can find yourself with a parasite called round worms. Roundworms cause the infection in the stomach called anisakiasis, and it can be painful.

2. Drinking infected water, such as in those streams and rivers that you are hiking by, is another source of parasites. One parasite from infected water is called Cryptosporidium. Another water-born parasite is called giardia, a protozoa which can cause an intestinal illness. There are more.

3. If that cook at a restaurant has not thoroughly washed his or her hands, then touches your food, remains of his feces with parasites within can be spread to you!

4. Parasites can even get in via your nose, mouth or your skin, thus the importance of taking those showers frequently.

5. Mosquitoes can be a source of parasites coming through your skin.

I'm purposely not getting into details about all the different names and kinds of parasites, as that might be incredibly boring to some readers. But if you want to see the names, Wiki has a good list here: *https://en.wikipedia.org/wiki/List_of_parasites_of_humans*

Symptoms of a Parasite Infection

It's not always easy to go by symptoms, as they may be silent. But with the variety of parasites, here are some of the symptoms that could be a clue, and you'll see that they are also clues of other issues! I'll mention testing below.

- diarrhea
- gas
- cramps
- stomach pain
- nausea
- lowered appetite
- anemia from blood loss
- achiness
- lowered nutrients
- weakness
- weight loss
- irritation around your anus or the vulva in women
- worsening of allergies
- fever

How to Test for Parasites

The Centers for Disease Control and Prevention[141] mention four to talk to your health provider about these:

---

[141] https://www.cdc.gov/parasites/references_resources/diagnosis.html

1. Stool testing is the premier way to find out if you have these nasty buggers feeding on you. The test will look for eggs and the parasites themselves.
2. If the stool didn't reveal the eggs or the parasites, another test is an Endoscopy (the use of a flexible tube with a light and camera to look into your gut) or a Colonoscopy (a scope inserted via the rectum)
3. Blood test, which is only looking for specific ones.
4. X-rays, MRI's or CAT scans—these look into your organs.

Treatment for Parasites

Remarkably, there are some natural treatments:

1. raw pumpkin seeds (green)[142] (especially against roundworms)
2. berberine[143]
3. black walnut[144]
4. garlic[145]
5. curcumin[146]
6. ginger[147] (which can be taken with the curcumin)

If needed, there's also an antibiotic called Metronidazole which targets many parasite varieties.

Here's a good article: *https://drjockers.com/type-parasites/*

[142] https://www.ncbi.nlm.nih.gov/pmc/articles/PMC5037735/
[143] https://www.ncbi.nlm.nih.gov/pubmed/10767672
[144] https://wellnessmama.com/257/black-walnut-hull-herb-profile/
[145] https://www.ncbi.nlm.nih.gov/pubmed/10594976
[146] https://www.ncbi.nlm.nih.gov/pubmed/26261481
[147] https://www.ncbi.nlm.nih.gov/pubmed/23583317

NOTES

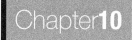

Chapter 10

Your Gut Part 2:
Dysbiosis, SIBO, Probiotics, Leaky Gut

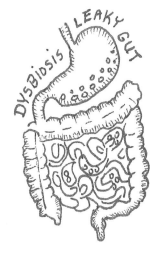

As explained in Chapter 9, having gut problems with Hashimoto's can be a real *pain in the gut*. The risk is too high that any gut problem can trigger flares like anxiety, pain, achiness, breathlessness, brain fog, feeling weak, fatigue, or anything that feels a bit off or suddenly hyper-like. Thus, the need to step back and do what it takes to treat any gut issue.

HASHIMOTO'S GUT PROBLEM #9:
Dysbiosis, aka an Imbalance of Your GI Tract Bacteria

Not all bacteria are bad! Some are good and needed.

Our lives start with beneficial gut bacteria even as newborns[148], especially from vaginal births. Those born via C-section may develop them over time.

Our digestive tract will eventually have billions upon billions of those beneficial microbes, aka bacteria or microbiome, to help with our immune system activity. That bacteria is also beneficial for good digestion, mental health, and vitamin production like the B's. In fact, our gut bacteria will outnumber our own cell count!

Research[149] shows that you can have
100 TRILLION little bacteria in your gut!

Gut bacteria are about "good diversity and balance", meaning not only a variety of good bacteria, but enough overall to outweigh potential bad bacteria and pathogens that could get in there. Simply put, the bad bacteria are opportunistic and can lead to disease without the diversity and a good number of good bacteria to counter them.

This bacterial gut community also has
connections to other parts of your body: i.e. the health
of your brain, kidneys, liver and lungs are also associated
with having diverse levels of good bacteria[150].

---

148 https://onlinelibrary.wiley.com/doi/full/10.1111/j.1365-2672.2007.03497.x
149 https://www.ncbi.nlm.nih.gov/pubmed/20192812
150 https://www.ncbi.nlm.nih.gov/pmc/articles/PMC4303825/

But for some of us, a problem can occur called dysbiosis, which is any change, increase or decrease, in the composition of the bacteria community.

Causes of Different Forms of Dysbiosis
(a change in one's gut bacteria)

- **Antibiotic use (can lower levels of good bacteria)** Though antibiotics can kill the bad bacteria, they will also lower your important good bacteria!

- **Genetics (certain mutations can cause lower levels of good bacteria)** For example, I have several homozygous (from both parents) variants/mutations in the FUT2 gene[151] [152], which means I never have strong amounts of bifidobacteria[153], a strong, health-promoting bacteria which are supposed to be large in quantity within the community of bacteria. Thus I need to supplement. And antibiotic use in me can promote overgrowth of gut pathogens, the bad guy bacteria, especially Clostridium difficile, because of FUT2. I found myself with too high levels of Clostridium once and treated it with monolaurin pellets. Monolaurin is from derived from lauric acid and is anti-bacteria.

- **Low bile levels (can cause excess bacteria)**[154] This is due to either sluggish liver production of bile or gallbladder stress/problems. Low bile may be what caused SIBO in me after doing a six-month high copper detox. I cover bile in #9 of this list.

- **Infections (can raise bad bacteria)** For example, research[155] shows that a hepatitis B viral infection can negatively alter your

[151] https://ndnr.com/gastrointestinal/fut2-secretor-status-effects-on-gut-health/
[152] http://www.beyondmthfr.com/fut2-genes-hidden-cause-leaky-gut-leaky-brain/
[153] https://www.ncbi.nlm.nih.gov/pmc/articles/PMC4908950/
[154] https://kresserinstitute.com/little-known-connection-leaky-gut-gluten-intolerance-gallblad-der-problems/
[155] https://www.ncbi.nlm.nih.gov/pmc/articles/PMC5483960/

gut bacteria. Another example: Influenza A virus[156] can alter gut bacteria. Salmonella[157] can disrupt the bacterial population.

- **Foods (poor nutrient foods can disturb the good bacteria balance)**[158] If you unfortunately like those packaged sticky buns, doughnuts and cinnamon rolls, be careful—they can contain emulsifiers which can negatively alter your gut bacteria.[159] There is also some evidence that GMO foods will negatively disturb your microbiome.[160]

- **Gum/tooth infection (can raise bad bacteria)** This can push bad bacteria into your stomach as you swallow—exactly what happened to me with an infected root canal, and I didn't know I had that infection for almost a year, yet had chronic stomach/digestive problems that made no sense to me at first.

More Causes of Unhealthy Changes in the Bacterial Community:

- poor pancreatic release of digestive enzymes
- slow movement of feces through the small intestine
- eating too much sugar which can feed even bad bacteria
- chronic stress
- exposure to pesticides
- alcoholism or simply drinking too much
- unprotected sex
- inflammatory bowel disease
- rheumatoid arthritis
- getting older

---

[156] https://www.ncbi.nlm.nih.gov/pmc/articles/PMC5763955/
[157] https://www.ncbi.nlm.nih.gov/pubmed/18160481
[158] https://www.ncbi.nlm.nih.gov/pmc/articles/PMC5872783/
[159] https://www.nature.com/articles/nature14232
[160] https://www.ncbi.nlm.nih.gov/pubmed/23224412

Symptoms of Dysbiosis Can Include:

- excessive gas
- bloating (when I once had SIBO, I'd get this badly after eating certain carbs, even good ones, before I realized why!)
- Headaches or migraines[161]
- stomach feeling upset / uncomfortable
- food sitting too long in the stomach
- diarrhea, sometimes alternating with constipation
- vaginal itching (candida)
- fatigue
- depression or anxiety
- brain fogginess
- bad breath
- urination difficulty
- getting a diagnosis of irritable bowel syndrome
- risk of Hashimoto's

Testing

Here are examples of tests to unveil what might be going on:

- *Comprehensive Stool Test[162]:* This comes from your doctor or you can order your own. It takes a look at bacteria, yeast and even parasites coming from your body into your feces.
- *Organic Acids Test (OAT) or the Organix® Dysbiosis Profile - Urine[163]:* The OAT you can order yourself such as by Great Plains, and it shows a bunch of info about you via your urine, in addition to gut issues. The Organix Dysbiosis profile is often ordered by your doctor.

---

[161] https://www.ncbi.nlm.nih.gov/pmc/articles/PMC5037083/
[162] https://www.greatplainslaboratory.com/comprehensive-stool-analysis/
[163] https://www.gdx.net/product/organix-dysbiosis-test-urine

- *Hydrogen breath test[164]:* This measures whether you have hydrogen present in your gut, which shouldn't be there. Thus, it's testing for issues like IBS (Irritable Bowel Syndrome) and SIBO (Small Intestinal Bacterial Overgrowth), plus other digestive problem related to food intolerances. Usually done by a doctor.
- *Intestinal Permeability Assessment[165]:* This tests your "small intestinal absorption and barrier function in the bowel", aka Leaky Gut. Doctors order this or there are some facilities where you can order it yourself.

Treatment

- Eating consistently healthier with plenty of greens, red and orange veggies, some low-glycemic fruits like berries, plus non-farmed fish and healthy meats—any of the latter that you know you tolerate. (Farmed fish are said to have food bathed in antibiotics or the fish themselves have disease.)
- Consuming fermented foods, which include kefir, greek yogurt, miso, sauerkraut or the fermented beverage called kombucha.
- Fiber-rich foods will feed your good bacteria.
- Lower your consumption of sugar and grains. They can be very triggering of Hashimoto's!
- Taking multiple strain probiotics with amounts of at least 1 to 10 billion CFU, along with prebiotics. Prebiotics are food for your good bacteria. Besides prebiotic supplements, food versions include bananas, apple skins, beans, dandelion greens, chicory root (I personally love chicory tea with cream and stevia.), onions, garlic, asparagus, leeks. Prebiotic fiber becomes fermented which feeds your beneficial bacteria.
- For bad cases and especially SIBO (Small Intestinal Bacterial

---

[164] https://en.wikipedia.org/wiki/Hydrogen_breath_test
[165] https://www.gdx.net/product/intestinal-permeability-assessment-urine

Overgrowth), there's an antibiotic (irony) called rifaximin (Xifaxan) that can help. And most literature states it doesn't have the bad side effects of other antibiotics.

All About SIBO: A More Well-Known Example of Dysbiosis on the "Excess" Side

Small Intestinal Bacterial Overgrowth (SIBO) is an example of an overgrowth of one's gut bacteria. It's about being in excess where it's not meant to be in excess: in the small intestine. In other words, most of your gut bacteria is supposed to be in your **large intestine and colon.** Those little bacteria play a role of helping you break down food, providing nutrients, and helping eliminate waste products.

But when the bacteria are in excess, they start feeding off carbs and starches in your **small intestine.** The result? Excess levels of hydrogen and/or methane. Gas! You then might feel very bloated after eating (I sure did when I had SIBO!), or having problems with burping, gas, or diarrhea.

Other reported symptoms of SIBO include pain in your joints, low levels of vitamins, smelly stools, rashes, fatigue, stomach cramping, and in some cases, constipation.

What Causes SIBO?
- problems in digestion
- slow movement through your GI tract, called a motility problem
- eating too much sugar or simple carbs
- low stomach acid
- drinking too much alcohol
- having Diabetes or Celiac
- any autoimmune disease
- aging
- low bile levels (this happened to me after a major detox of heavy metals)

How to Diagnose SIBO

A great way to diagnose is via a hydrogen and/or methane breath test, also called a lactulose breath test. This test can be done in your own home. Lactulose is a carbohydrate and is swallowed in a drink. You then breathe into an analyzer every 20 minutes for three hours. High levels of hydrogen produced by the fermentation of unabsorbed carbohydrates will help diagnose SIBO and is usually the most common high result. A lower amount of SIBO patients will have high levels of methane, and some are positive for both hydrogen and methane.[166]

There's also a glucose breath test, but studies show that the above lactose breath test gives better results in diagnosis.[167]

Bloating is the most common SIBO symptom that leads to be being tested.

Treatment of SIBO

There are many ways to treat. I personally chose to use natural herbs and products that act like antibiotics, such as garlic oil capsules, berberine, oregano oil capsules, and olive leaf extract. I took two of the latter four for a few weeks (several of each), then the other two for another few weeks (several of each). I also incorporated the Specific Carbohydrate Diet[168], i.e. I was eating free of grains, sugar, starches and especially unprocessed foods of any kind.

[166] https://www.ncbi.nlm.nih.gov/pmc/articles/PMC5660265/
[167] https://www.ncbi.nlm.nih.gov/pmc/articles/PMC5660265/
[168] https://scdlifestyle.com/about-the-scd-diet/

> **Warning:** I personally did the herbal treatment too long!! That caused candida overgrowth. So I strongly recommend to learn from others, which I didn't do first. There are good SIBO websites to search for and read on the internet.

There is also a good and safe antibiotic called Rifaximin[169] to use against SIBO instead of the natural ones I used. I honestly wish I had gone the Rifaximin route, but the natural route works well, too.

Also recommended is to eat smaller meals to enable faster digestion and movement of food.

Why Taking Probiotics (beneficial bacteria) Can Help Those with a Bad Bacteria Buildup

1. Strong levels of good gut bacteria help counter and crowd out the bad opportunistic bacteria.
2. Good bacteria promote better conversion of thyroid hormone T4 to the active thyroid hormone T3.[170]
3. Good bacteria has a positive effect on your brain's ability to think and remember.
4. If for any reason an antibiotic is needed, probiotics taken between doses and especially after the full course help replenish the positive bacterial community.
5. Probiotics like bifida infantis can help relieve symptoms from IBS.[171]
6. Probiotics/good bacteria communicate with the immune system to do its job better.

---

[169] https://www.ncbi.nlm.nih.gov/pmc/articles/PMC5299503/

[170] https://kresserinstitute.com/gut-microbes-thyroid-whats-connection/

[171] http://citeseerx.ist.psu.edu/viewdoc/download?doi=10.1.1.474.2780&rep=rep1&type=pdf

Probiotic Strains to Consider

In some ways, there is no probiotic right for all people who find they need to crowd out bad bacteria or replenish their good bacteria after having dysbiosis issues. But below is a list of typical beneficial strains and what they may help.

Most people choose multiple-strain probiotics and also rotate versions. It's not about taking just one of the below, though for me, I need bifido's for the rest of my life.

1. Bifido's (Bifidobacterium)[172] which are mainly in the large intestine. These little ones can help your immune system, digestion, relieve bloating, prevent or treat colon cancer, relieve symptoms of inflammatory bowel disease, help treat eczema, and more.

Examples are:

- Bifidobacterium bifidum (reduces E. coli and h-pylori infections, reduces acute diarrhea, treats irritable bowel infections)
- Bifidobacterium breve (suppresses fat deposits, improves cholesterol and glucose levels)
- Bifidobacterium infantis (helps irritable bowel and reduces gas, anti-inflammatory)
- Bifidobacterium lactis (anti-tumor growth, enhances better immune function, helps vitamin and mineral gut absorption, improves digestion)
- Bifidobacterium longum (helps prevent infections, lessons symptoms of a cold or flu, produces B1, B2, B6, and vitamin K)

2. Lacto's (Lactobacillus)[173] These can help treat diarrhea or constipation, improve vaginal health, treat or prevent the skin

---

[172] https://www.ncbi.nlm.nih.gov/pmc/articles/PMC4908950/
[173] https://en.wikipedia.org/wiki/Lactobacillus

disorder eczema, can lower the toxicity of candida…and more.

Examples are:

- Lactobacillus acidophilus (help reduces high cholesterol, improve irritable bowels, can reduce allergy symptoms)

- Lactobacillus brevis (helps support natural killer (NK) cells, promotes better mood, used to make wines tastier)

- Lactobacillus bilgaricus (lowers intestinal pH to halt bacterial growth, helps ferment yogurt, cheeses, beer, and wine)

- Lactobacillus casei (antimicrobial, helps modulate immune system, improves intestinal lining)

- Lactobacillus DDS-1 (improves side effects of lactose intolerance, modulates immune system, shortens respiratory infection along with bifido's)

- Lactobacillus delbruecki (anti-inflammatory, used in yogurt starter with Streptococcus thermophilus, treats ulcerative colitis)

- Lactobacillus helveticus (can lower anxiety, anger and depression, can help lower cortisol)

- Lactobacillus lactis (can inhibit cancer cells, used in buttermilk and cheese production)

- Lactobacillus plantarum (strong antioxidant, helps prevent leaky gut)

- Lactobacillus reuteri (strong anti-inflammatory cytokines, prevents leaky gut)

- Lactobacillus rhamnosus (treats bacterial vaginosis, prevents diarrhea)

- Lactobacillus salivarius (helps manage pancreatic necrosis, lowers gas from irritable bowels, suppresses bad bacteria)

Plus…

3. **Streptococcus thermophilus**[174]: found in yogurt, helps break down lactose, can reduce diarrhea from antibiotic use, more

4. **Saccharomyces boulardii**[175]: not really a bacteria, but a non-pathogenic yeast used as a probiotic that helps counter inflammation from gastrointestinal diseases, decreases Crohn's caused leaky gut, good against h-pylori and Clostridium difficile infection, against diarrhea, and more.

Experts recommend taking probiotics for up to six months to repopulate an injured microbiotic community, then reduce and enjoy fermented foods like a Kombucha drink, yogurt, and even pickles.

> I am a Greek Yogurt lover, which has the good bacteria lactobacillus bulgaricus and streptococcus thermophilus. I put ½ cup or more in a bowl, add green pumpkin seeds, a few dried non-sugar cherries, a little vanilla plus stevia. YUM.

How to Prevent a Dysbiosis Problem in the First Place

Dysbiosis in general might be prevented with the following:
- the right amount of stomach acid / gastric acid
- good movements (intestinal motility) in the small intestine to your anus (magnesium helps)
- taking digestive enzymes
- having good dental hygiene
- avoiding excess alcohol
- taking betaine, since stomach acid directly destroys bad bacteria, besides lowering the pH value in the small intestine. [176]

[174] https://en.wikipedia.org/wiki/Streptococcus_thermophilus
[175] https://www.ncbi.nlm.nih.gov/pmc/articles/PMC3296087/
[176] https://www.ncbi.nlm.nih.gov/pmc/articles/PMC4566455/

HASHIMOTO'S GUT PROBLEM #10:
Leaky Gut

Who would've guessed that those intestines we all learned about in science class would leak! But they can.

Leaky gut, aka "intestinal permeability", does have some controversy. It's *"does leaky gut cause certain conditions"*, or *"do the conditions cause the leaky gut"*? The answer? It may be both ways... but there seems to be more emphasis in literature and studies as to what leaky gut can cause.

> Leaky gut refers to having bacteria, viruses, toxins, and even undigested food particles leak through what should be a protected intestinal mucosal lining, but has become compromised. This predisposes those with an autoimmune tendency to get worse.

In other words, as part of the immune system, the mucus lining in the intestines is supposed to be the first line of defense against having the latter substances leak through. Conversely, the lining should be tight enough to only allow nutrients through.

But when that lining becomes permeable / leaky, and particles get through where they shouldn't be, the immune system is going to naturally activate to attempt to neutralize those particles...along with causing inflammation.

And as the invaders continue to come through, the immune system just might become overreactive like those 20 hands slapping a single mosquito... overkill. Then one's own healthy cells could start to be attacked in those susceptible, i.e. autoimmunity and more inflammation develops! [177]

---

[177] https://link.springer.com/article/10.1007/s12016-011-8291-x

How Leaky Gut Can Affect Your Liver, Gallbladder and Bile Ducts

If one has a leaky gut, gut bad bacteria can sneak its way through and into your blood stream. Thus, there can be...

- an immune system reaction, or
- an autoimmune overreaction.

And the latter creates inflammation. That inflammation can affect the biliary system (the bile transport system from the liver's production, to storage by the gallbladder, to problems with the bile ducts.)

One article proposes that 1) infection leads to 2) leaky gut and 3) leaky gut leads to Hashimoto's[178], i.e. Hashi's is the result of a leaky gut.

Proposed Causes of Leaky Gut

- candida[179]
- allergies to certain foods you eat
- inflammation causing foods
- SIBO (small intestinal bacteria overgrowth)
- celiac disease
- crohn's disease/ inflammatory bowel disease
- excess use of aspirin, ibuprofen, or acetaminophen[180]
- alcoholism[181]
- excessive exercise[182]
- parasites[183]
- inflammation in the digestive tract

---

[178] https://justinhealth.com/hashimotos-infection-connection/
[179] https://www.yeastinfection.org/yeast-infections-and-leaky-gut-syndrome/
[180] https://www.ncbi.nlm.nih.gov/pubmed/29094594
[181] https://www.ncbi.nlm.nih.gov/pmc/articles/PMC2614138/
[182] https://www.sciencedaily.com/releases/2017/06/170607085452.htm
[183] https://drjockers.com/type-parasites/

Dr. Bill Rawls[184] suggests three causes of leaky gut:

    1) lectins, gluten, and excessive carbs

    2) chronic stress

    3) toxins

Another research states that the autoimmune problem of Celiac can cause leaky gut, whereas removing gluten seems to reverse it.[185]

Even back in 1999, research showed a connection between leaky gut and the autoimmune Crohn's disease.[186]

Research also shows a connection of leaky gut to irritable bowel syndrome[187]

The following are stated to be connected to a leaky gut:

- inflammatory and infectious bowel diseases
- chronic inflammatory arthritis
- acne
- psoriasis
- itchy rash (dermatitis herpetiformis) associated with celiac
- eczema
- urticaria
- irritable bowel syndrome
- AIDS
- chronic fatigue syndromes or just fatigue
- chronic hepatitis
- chronic pancreatitis
- cystic fibrosis
- pancreatic carcinoma
- candida

---

[184] https://rawlsmd.com/health-articles/the-leaky-gut-epidemic-modern-causes-natural-solutions

[185] https://www.ncbi.nlm.nih.gov/pmc/articles/PMC3458511/

[186] https://link.springer.com/article/10.1007/s11894-999-0023-5

[187] https://www.karger.com/Article/Abstract/333083

Leaky gut might equal a red flag for developing inflammation and even worse, for developing autoimmune diseases. Conversely, autoimmune-caused inflammation, or any chronic inflammation, may cause leaky gut! Either way, it's not something you want.

Symptoms of Leaky Gut

Dr. Leo Galland[188] lists these symptoms of leaky gut:

- arthritis
- allergies
- depression
- eczema
- hives
- psoriasis
- chronic fatigue syndrome
- fibromyalgia

Check out one of his wonderful articles: *http://www.mdheal.org/leakygut.htm*

How to test for leaky gut

1. Genova Diagnostics has an Intestinal Permeability Assessment[189] that can be ordered by your doctor.

2. Another test is called the Lactulose/Mannitol Test.[190] There are facilities where you can order your own (do a search on your laptop or computer), or ask your doctor about it.

3. Cyrex Laboratories[191] has a blood test called Intestinal Antigenic Permeability Screen[192].

---

[188] https://www.metsol.com/assets/sites/2/Do-you-have-leaky-gut-syndrome.pdf
[189] https://www.gdx.net/product/intestinal-permeability-assessment-urine
[190] https://www.ncbi.nlm.nih.gov/pubmed/10902869
[191] https://www.cyrexlabs.com/CyrexTestsArrays
[192] https://store.thedr.com/product/array-2-intestinal-antigenic-permeability-screen/

What to do about Leaky Gut?

Here are a variety of suggestions:

1. **Lower stress:** Find ways to reduce stress in your life. It could be meditation, taking deep breaths, sleeping enough hours, doing activities you love, pursuing a relaxing and fun hobby, having healthy people in your life and limiting toxic people, find videos that make you laugh…

> Once, when I was under a LOT of stress from a job, I made a point on Sunday nights to watch funny shows on TV that I knew would make me belly laugh.

2. **Avoid problematic foods:** Identify and avoid foods that cause you problems or reactions. *This is a very important step.*

3. **Lower antibodies:** Do whatever it takes to lower an autoimmune response, since it promotes inflammation. When you get to Chapter 16, you'll see all the way patients are lowering their antibodies.

4. **Take Gut healing supplements:**
   - *L-glutamine amino acid* - helps produce mucus in the lining
   - *Fiber* - helps feed the bifidobacteria, which helps heal leaky gut and also pushes bad bacteria out
   - *Monolaurin* - kills the bacteria or fungus trying to come through one's leaky gut. I use monolaurin pellets if I have a bacterial or vital infection. They usually come with a scoop, and you can drink them down.
   - *Lemon juice in water* - provides acid to the stomach, helps kill bad guys that are leaking through
   - *Curcumin* - very anti-inflammatory. I usually take far more than the bottle says to take, but make sure you are tolerant of it first.
   - *Quercetin* to counter high histamine which causes inflammation. Buckwheat tea is stated to have high amounts of quercitin.

5. **Eat foods that promote good gut bacteria** Yogurt, pickles yogurt and kefir are a few examples.

6. **Limit your intake of alcohol and sugar**. Moderation or abstinence is healthier.

7. **Treat inflammation and the cause**. There are great supplements out there like curcumin, ginger, etc. I personally have to take several caps of curcumin morning and night to control inflammation. Consider moderation or avoidance of inflammation-causing foods like dairy, sugar or processed foods.

8. **Natural Desiccated Thyroid**[193] **or T4/T3 for thyroid meds**. Learn to be optimal, not just "on" them. Read the updated revision STTM book[194] along with this one. Check out the Stop the Thyroid Madness website[195]. The right meds will help bring stomach acid up and lower problems caused by not correctly treating one's hypo-thyroid state, which includes hypothyroid-induced inflammation.

9. **Natural Desiccated Thyroid**[196] **or T4/T3 for thyroid meds**. Learn to be optimal, not just "on" them. Read the updated revision STTM book[197] along with this one. Check out the Stop the Thyroid Madness website[198]. The right meds will help bring up stomach acid and lower problems caused by one's hypothyroid state, which includes hypothyroid-induced inflammation.

10. **Coconut Charcoal supplements to bind and remove toxins**, suggests Dr. Jill Carnahan.[199] She also suggests the use of the probiotic Lactobacillus rhamnosus GG. Research confirms the use of Lactobacillus rhamnosus for gut lining.[200]

---

[193] http://stopthethyroidmadness.com/natural-thyroid-101
[194] http://laughinggrapepublishing.com
[195] http://stopthethyroidmadness.com
[196] http://stopthethyroidmadness.com/natural-thyroid-101
[197] http://laughinggrapepublishing.com
[198] http://stopthethyroidmadness.com
[199] https://www.jillcarnahan.com/2018/01/07/9-simple-steps-to-heal-leaky-gut-syndrome-fast/
[200] https://www.ncbi.nlm.nih.gov/pmc/articles/PMC3864899/

TIDBITS

■ In reference to leaky gut, a 2011 study proposed that leaky gut might cause diabetes, just as closing what should be tight gaps in the intestinal barrier could be a good treatment for diabetes.[201]

■ Research shows that leaky gut in older adults predicts their inflammation burden[202].

---

[201] https://www.ncbi.nlm.nih.gov/pmc/articles/PMC3864899/
[202] https://academic.oup.com/innovateage/article/2/suppl_1/93/5170479

NOTES

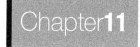
The Problem of Stress on Your Adrenals

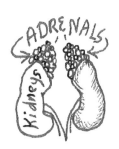

In 2002, when I began the patient-to-patient movement I later termed Stop the Thyroid Madness (after I myself suffered miserably from a poor treatment for nearly two decades), it didn't take long to notice that a large body of patients in an early group I owned were reporting symptoms that didn't just seem like typical thyroid or autoimmune issues. Some did, but a lot were beyond that.

So, we did some reading and research, even talking to patients with Addison's disease—another autoimmune situation where the adrenals were being attacked. And some of the symptoms matched, even though no one in the group had Addison's.

It didn't take long to figure out that many thyroid patients were finding themselves with high cortisol, or low cortisol, or mixed highs and lows. The adrenals were stressed!

And Hashimoto's patients were especially susceptible to seeing stressed adrenals with the additional stress of their autoimmune issues (emotional and physical) and flares.

Let's look at some symptoms that patients with adrenal problems reported over the years, and still do[203]. You can have some, but not others. Some are more based on low cortisol; others can be about high cortisol. **Recognize any of these stressed adrenal/low cortisol symptoms?**

anxiety	fatigue
feelings of panic	fast heartrate
shaky	heart stress
easily defensive	heart palps
paranoid	low back pain
lack of patience	bright light discomfort
easily irritated	noise discomfort
easy to anger	brain issues
hyper sensitive	confusion
over-reactive	headaches
argumentative	feeling bad
low stress tolerance	morning unrefreshed
people avoidant	insomnia
jumpy/jittery	waking up nighttime
nausea with stress	low blood sugar
feeling hyper	high blood sugar
weight gain	high blood pressure
allergy increase	worsening Hashi's flares

Once symptoms were recognized, patients were then, and are now, doing a **24-hour saliva cortisol test**[204] *(https://tinyurl.com/saliva-cortisol)* to see exactly what is going, especially since some symptoms can be similar with high cortisol or with low cortisol, thus treatment is different.

---

[203] https://stopthethyroidmadness.com/adrenal-info/symptoms-low-cortisol/
[204] http://stopthethyroidmadness.com/saliva-cortisol

Why saliva testing over blood—the latter which some doctors still tend to wrongly recommend? Two reasons:

> 1) Blood is a one-time test, and that's not enough to understand what is going on. Saliva measures cortisol levels are four key times in your waking period, which is important.
>
> 2) Blood is mostly measuring bound, unusable cortisol—80% or more. We need to know what is unbound and being used, which saliva tests.
> http://stopthethyroidmadness.com/saliva-cortisol

We also learned, as has been compiled on the website Stop the Thyroid Madness, that the results have nothing to do with falling anywhere in those ranges. It's about where in the range they fall[205]. Use this page: *https://stopthethyroidmadness.com/lab-values*

Doing saliva testing also revealed that results were not matching the levels of cortisol in those who didn't have a cortisol problem at all.[206]

In healthy situations, what are my adrenals supposed to be doing for me?

Your little but protective adrenal glands (located on your lower back, on top of your kidneys) are meant to respond to stress to help you deal with stress.

The adrenals respond to stress by releasing both extra cortisol and adrenaline.

---

[205] http://stopthethyroidmadness.com/lab-values
[206] http://stopthethyroidmadness.com/lab-values

Adrenaline, also called epinephrine,
is released to sharpen your brain and senses to what is going on.
It will increase your heart rate, which increases blood flow and
stimulates more energy. It helps you breathe in more oxygen. It
gets your brain moving and your pupils wider.

Cortisol is released to bring your blood sugar levels up—the latter
to give you more energy to deal with stress better. Cortisol also
goes up in response to one's autoimmune-caused inflammation—
trying to control damage caused by that inflammation.

But your adrenals aren't releasing adrenaline and cortisol on their
own accord. They are messaged to do so by the pituitary gland's
release of the messenger hormone called the Adrenocorticotropic
hormone, aka the ACTH. The ACTH is going to knock on the door
of your adrenals to tell them to respond to what is going on with the
release of adrenaline and cortisol.

Where the Trouble Begins

The adrenal trouble you can find yourself in is due to the chronic
nature of having Hashimoto's disease—ongoing inflammation from
the attack, a variety of environmental triggers which make your
Hashi's worse (certain foods, toxin exposure, smoking, excess alcohol
and more), chronic gut issues (See Chapters 9 and 10), any infections,
and even life stresses. And when any problems are ongoing, the risk
increases that cortisol can go up and stay up for too long. You might
also notice hyper-like symptoms like anxiety and shakiness from
high adrenaline.

Prolonged high cortisol is especially problematic.

Chronically high cortisol can cause some of the following:

- weight gain
- fatigue
- rising reverse T3 (makes hypothyroid worse)
- high free T3 (called pooling)
- nausea
- pimples or acne
- high blood sugar
- sleep problems
- weakness
- irritability
- high blood pressure
- more digestive/ gastrointestinal problems

This is why it's ludicrous if anyone says to you *"Let your Hashimoto's run its course."* Nope. Nope.

In fact, that high cortisol will cause either a) your natural production of T4 (the thyroid storage hormone), or b) treatment with synthetic T4, to convert to increasing levels of the inactive thyroid hormone called reverse T3 (RT3). And the higher RT3 goes, the lower the active thyroid hormone called T3 goes, since the RT3 is hogging the cell receptors. Cell receptors are molecules that receive thyroid hormones, allowing them to anchor on the cells.

And all the latter that makes you even more hypo.

Why T4-only medications can also push cortisol up

Years of patient experiences and observations have taught us that those who are put on synthetic T4-only medications like Synthroid, Levothyroxine, Eltroxin, Oroxine, etc. have a risk of seeing their cortisol go up and up.

Why? The body is alarmed.

We are not meant to live for T4 alone, a storage hormone. A healthy body makes five thyroid hormones, not just one[207]: T4, T3, T2, T1 and calcitonin. T4 will be converting to T3, yes. T3 is the active thyroid hormone which makes us feel better. But you also get direct T3. The latter is missing when you are put on nothing but T4.

Yes, some feel pretty good at first on T4. It's converting to the active T3. But it appears to be only a matter of time that depending solely on T4 to convert to T3 will mess up...as we have observed in ourselves and each other for decades. Then, you can notice hypothyroid symptoms creeping up, which can include depression, hair loss, dry skin, rising blood pressure or cholesterol, aches and pains, the need to nap, heart issues, bone loss, anxiety, or other problems that you may not know are connected to being on a poor treatment.

And in addition to those hypothyroid symptoms on T4, cortisol and adrenaline can start to go up due to the alarm of a poor treatment... sooner or later.

How high cortisol eventually falls off the cliff to low

Eventually, the body is not going to like that ongoing high cortisol. It's problematic to your health and well-being. So, your body is going to cause the high cortisol to start a fall to low cortisol.

Dr. Lena D. Edwards calls this low cortisol state "hypocortisolism" in the last Chapter of the Stop the Thyroid Madness II book with chapters contributed by certain medical professionals. The last chapter by Dr. Edwards goes into excellent detail about the mechanisms behind high falling into low cortisol. Highly recommended.

Many of the symptoms listed on the previous page are true for low

---

[207] http://stopthethyroidmadness.com/t4-only-meds-dont-work

cortisol.   And with low cortisol, you have problems raising better thyroid meds like desiccated thyroid, or synthetic T4 with synthetic T3, or straight T3.

The problem of increasing thyroid meds with low cortisol

For one, the free T3 starts going high, because without enough cortisol, T3 will hang out in the blood and not make it to the cells. Or you can see increased anxiety, or shakiness, or a fast heartrate, or heart palps.   Sadly, because doctors may not understand the low cortisol (or high cortisol) problem when raising better thyroid meds, they blame the medications. In actuality, the better thyroid meds are "revealing" the problem---a cortisol problem.

Not a pretty picture, is it?

Patient Reported Information for a Cortisol Problem

Please understand that the following information is just that— information as experienced by patients over the years.   It is not personal medical advice. Work with your doctor.

1. If there's a suspicion of an adrenal problem, there are some insightful Discovery Steps that can reveal a potential adrenal problem here: *http://stopthethyroidmadness.com/adrenal-info*

2. If symptoms and answers to the important Discovery Steps point to an adrenal problem, patients know that doing a 24-hour cortisol saliva test has given them more precise information rather than blood. Blood is measuring mostly bound cortisol, of which 80% or more is bound. It's also only one time of the day. Saliva measures useable and unbound cortisol. Here is an affiliated example of a saliva test that can be done in your own home: *https:// tinyurl.com/saliva-cortisol.* The Discovery Steps mentioned

in #1 on the previous page can also potentially reveal an aldosterone problem,[208] another steroid produced in the adrenals, i.e. via the pupil test, and especially via the blood pressure sit-down/stand up test. It appears that around 50% of patients with a cortisol problem also have low aldosterone. More about that here: *http://stopthethyroidmadness.com/aldosterone*

3. We also compare the results to where patients fall who don't have a problem. i.e. it's not about those too-broad ranges. This page shows where people fall who don't have a cortisol or aldosterone problem to compare to: *https://stopthethyroidmadness.com/lab-values* All based on years and years of observations. Teach this to your doctor.

4. Here is information based on years of patient experiences with the saliva cortisol results to use in working with a doctor, and you may have to work to find an open-minded doctor. This information is not presented to use on your own. I t is expected that any reader takes responsibility and works with the guidance of a doctor.

    a. **If saliva results show minor to moderate low results three or more times in a row,** as revealed by comparing to what's on the Lab Values page, patients found out they need cortisol supplementation like adrenal cortex, 50 mg capsules, during those low times. Why? We can't get out of our hypothyroid state if cortisol is low, since cortisol is needed for thyroid hormones to get to the cells. And being hypothyroid is a major contributor to a cortisol problem in the first place, as well as other stresses.

    b. **If saliva results show four quite low results towards the bottom of each range,** patients follow their doctor's

---

[208] http://stopthethyroidmadness.com/aldosterone

guidance and rule out Addison's disease, first, or even hypopituitary (failure of the pituitary gland in releasing the ACTH messenger hormone). Patients are then usually put on prescription hydrocortisone (common name is Cortef, but there are others) in working with their doctor. Starting dose for women is 25 mgs total, spaced four hours apart starting in the morning with 10 mg, then every four hours in descending doses to equal 25. Starting dose for men is 30 mg, starting on 12 mg in the morning and then the rest spaced out the next three four-hour intervals in descending doses, to equal 30.

c. **If saliva results show two highs and two lows, each in a row,** patients first work on lowering those two highs. There are many good cortisol-lowering supplements patients use, like holy basil (if they tolerate basil products), or zinc (if copper isn't too high, as zinc will start a detox), or phosphatidyl serine. Patients take them one hour before a high as revealed by a cortisol saliva test. Lowering the highs eventually helps raise the lows.

d. **If results are like a see-saw, such as low, high, low, high or vice versa**, patients found it means the adrenals are in an early stressed stage, and using adaptogens[209] several times a day helps reverse that. See footnote link below.

There are more excellent adrenal and cortisol details in working with your doctor, found in Chapter 6 of the updated revised book *Stop the Thyroid Madness: A Patient Revolution Against Decades of Inferior Thyroid Treatment.* It also applies to Adrenal Cortex.

---

[209] http://stopthethyroidmadness.com/adaptogens

Can adrenal stress be prevented in the first place?

Yes, if you see that you have family members with autoimmune issues, even if you don't have high thyroid antibodies, or catch your antibodies going up soon enough, there are ways to lower the risk. Lowering the risk starts with the same strategies that patients in the throes of Hashimoto's help themselves from flares. Namely, work on lowering stress in your life and pay attention if you are already having reactions to certain foods and eliminate them. Use "supportive" immune supplements like Vitamin C, B-vitamins, Elderberry, etc. Consider being on a variety of probiotics or eating fermented foods. Avoid exposure to toxins outside or inside. Keep your vitamin D levels optimal (over 50 or even 60-80). You'll see all sorts of strategies that patients implement in the rest of the chapters of this book.

Remember: all in this Chapter is simply information based on years of patient reports and experiences. The information is to be used in working with a doctor. This is not about recommending you to do it on your own.

Bottom line: It's relatively common to see many, but not all, Hashimoto's patients end up with a cortisol problem due to all the autoimmune triggers, flares, stress, inflammation, infections, being hypothyroid without treatment, or simply being on T4 meds. But it's all very treatable.

TIDBITS

- The bad thing about chronic stress of any kind is that it will first activate your immune system (which isn't great if you have autoimmune Hashimoto's) then will activate the release of cortisol.

NOTES

Chapter 12

Why Do Hashimoto's Patients Go Years **without a Diagnosis?**

Yes, reports by a large body of patients imply that the majority of Hashi's patients go years before they find out what they have had all that time. It can be 5+ years, 10+ years, 20+ years, 30+ years before the important autoimmune component diagnosis is made.

What seems obvious is that too many patients are walking through the first two stages of Hashi's, as seen in

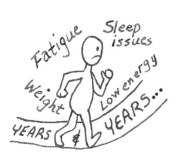

Chapter 3, without awareness, i.e. *1. The Calm Before the Storm; Predisposition* and 2. *The Rise of Antibodies: Silent for some, Obvious for others.*

But many also appear to be walking into the third stage without awareness of the cause of their problems, i.e. *3. The Growth and Onslaught of the Anti-Thyroid Army.* The thyroid is being cruelly attacked to the point of permanent damage and hypothyroidism setting in!

And for some, even this thyroid damage stage can go on for years without a diagnosis of Hashimoto's disease to explain it. Then patients are put on an inadequate way to treat their hypothyroidism: T4-only meds like Synthroid, Levothyroxine, Eltroxin, Oroxine etc. Yes, some do better than others at first. But forcing the body to live for conversion alone to T3, which is what T4 is about, will eventually cause growing problems.

Then comes the unintended gaslighting by uninformed doctors, family or friends when you talk about your symptoms. Gaslighting means comments by someone which cast doubt on your reality.

Recognize any of these gaslighting comments below?

You just need to exercise more and eat less...
This is all happening because you're a mother/parent...
You are simply working too hard and stressed...
You are just getting older...
You are depressed...
You're too nervous...
You're too driven...
You are a hypochondriac...
You just need to see a therapist or psychiatrist...
Maybe you have "this disease" or "that condition"...
You're complaining too much...
You are a difficult patient...
All you need to do is nap more, do yoga, meditate...

Summary of 6 explanations for failing to get a diagnosis of Hashimoto's

1) Any of the above statements made to you.

The term gaslighting refers to any well-meaning, but inaccurate judgments or comments said to you that end up making you question the reality of what your own observations or symptoms! Unfortunately, being gaslighted is very common with certain doctors, too.

2) Patient resistance

Though not as common a cause, some patients do report just pushing through their busy life and not approaching their doctor through the years, in spite of growing symptoms. They might be called "health deniers". (I can be like that. lol). i.e. "I was too busy to find out."

3) Lack of understanding or education

Though patients know that some of their family members or recent ancestors had certain health conditions, they simply didn't understand…

a) the autoimmune component of what some family members have or had

b) the genetic risk of seeing the same in themselves

c) ways to put Hashimoto's into remission

4) A doctor's failure to do antibodies testing

This turns out to be the most commonly expressed reason by patients to explain why they have gone so many years with Hashimoto's signs and symptoms, yet no diagnosis. Says one patient: *"I've seen a handful of doctors over the years, but labs for thyroid antibodies were never ordered, nor was the autoimmune component suggested to me!"*.

In a few reported cases, one antibody was ordered by their doctor (frequently the anti-TPO) and it was fine. Yet, if the other antibody had been tested, aka anti-thyroglobulin, it might be high! Without both, some cases of Hashimoto's can be missed. This is why Stop the Thyroid Madness reports that it's crucial to have BOTH antibodies tested, not just one.

This is also the area where many Hashi's patients are put on T4-only based on their symptoms, but it's proven repeatedly by years of patient experiences to be the worst way to treat one's hypothyroidism.[210] Or they are put on Natural Desiccated Thyroid or T4/T3, both far superior ways to treat hypothyroidism, but held to low doses and not allowed to be optimal.

5) Antibodies revealed, but the doctor's advice was similar to "Let it run its course" or "Nothing can be done".

Letting Hashimoto's run its course is akin to saying …

- *Continue to do nothing.*
- *Continue to let the antibodies go up.*
- *Continue to have other problems like high cortisol, low cortisol, low iron, low B12, low vitamin D, rising cholesterol, rising blood pressure, depression, anxiety and a host of other symptoms related to the continued attack and slow death of the thyroid. And to the contrary, patients have realized there is plenty that can be done, which this book is about!*

6) Antibodies revealed, but doctor nixes treatment until the TSH is higher

Nothing is more messed up than doctors who have made the TSH lab test like it's been dictated from a "Almighty, Omniscient, and Supreme God of Lab Testing". Yet, informed patients know that this pituitary hormone lab test can take years before it rises high enough to reveal the problem going on all that time…if it even rises!![211] I personally had a dear friend who had been clearly hypothyroid for 15 years, plus now had low cortisol, and her TSH was never higher than the low 2's…very "in range". All she could do all those years, while doctors only tested her TSH, was soldier through it as a single mother.

---

[210] http://stopthethyroidmadness.com/t4-only-meds-dont-work
[211] http://stopthethyroidmadness.com/tsh-why-its-useless

7) Antibodies revealed, but no guidance about your gut health, about triggers including what you eat, or how to better treat one's hypothyroid state.

The gut and trigger information in this book will now help. For the best way to treat one's hypothyroidism, how to read labs, how to treat related conditions caused by the hypothyroid state, I strongly recommend the website *http://stopthethyroidmadness.com/* and the Stop the Thyroid Madness books—links for those books are on the site.

First Symptoms; Subsequent Symptoms

Starting on the next page are the words of Hashimoto's patients--a compilation of their very first symptoms, which they feel initially revealed that something was amiss.

First symptoms have three properties:
1) They will vary between individuals.
2) They can be singular first signs, or multiple signs.
3) They can be followed by even more symptoms.

For example, if one person's first noted symptom was fatigue, they might have subsequent symptoms of weight gain or sleep problems. Conversely, if another patient's first symptom was about sleep problems, they might have subsequent symptoms of fatigue or anxiety.

The age of first symptoms will vary. Some report seeing them in their childhood. Some report them first in their teenage years. Some report seeing them in young adulthood, middle adulthood, or pre- or post-menopausal. Adulthood in general is the most common time frame for first signs.

Identify with any of the below first signs when looking back at when your Hashimoto's might have been showing itself?

Fatigue

This is the most common response by patients as the first sign that they had Hashimoto's disease, whether they recognized the autoimmune problem back then or not.

Fatigue by patients is expressed as follows:

- fatigue was constant
- fatigue was debilitating
- fatigue that wore me down
- it was sudden
- was unable to live my life due to my fatigue
- felt totally exhausted
- was needing constant naps
- couldn't keep eyes open when driving
- couldn't keep my eyes open in school
- would fall asleep watching TV
- heavy eyelids
- sleepy, sleepy
- felt extreme lethargy
- very tired
- low energy
- too tired participate in sports/jogging/running
- having to nap after regular chores or showering
- had no motivation suddenly/used to be the opposite

Sleep Issues

Another very common first sign of having Hashimoto's.

The sleep issues were expressed by patients as follows:

- insomnia
- couldn't stay asleep at night
- sleeping too many hours at night
- sleeping towards noon or early afternoon
- poor quality sleep
- sleeping many hours and still feeling exhausted
- waking up in the middle of night
- waking up needing more oxygen
- night sweating
- no amount sleep would take away the exhaustion
- waking/sleeping/waking/sleeping
- constant drowsiness
- trouble driving long distances
- napping all the time
- constant sleeping in teens
- constant sleeping in my 20s (or 30s, or 40s, or onward in age)

Weight Gain

Another very common early sign.

It's been expressed by patients as follows:

- slow but steady gain
- very fast gain within a short time
- massive gain
- 25+ lbs, 50+ lbs, 100+ lbs
- looked pregnant but wasn't
- couldn't fit in my jeans anymore
- gaining in spite of eating right

Weight Loss

Though not as common, weight loss has been a clear first sign for some, probably due to the hyper swing of the attack.

Lack of Energy

- just didn't have the umpff suddenly
- body felt heavy all the time
- ran out of steam a lot
- couldn't jog as long as I used to
- couldn't walk very far
- couldn't complete daily housework
- had to shorten grocery shopping
- didn't have the energy to play with my kids

Brain problems

- brain fog
- ability to think was slower
- couldn't recall certain words
- memory was suddenly poor
- felt muddled
- felt foggy
- wasn't able to concentrate

Hair Issues

- loss of hair
- noticeable thinning/ponytail was thinner
- falling out in clumps in shower
- drier hair than it used to be
- frizzy where it had never been before
- messy looking all the time
- breaking hair

- graying early
- losing eyebrows
- thinning eyelashes

Coughing

- dry cough
- feeling like something always in my throat
- throat tickling

Constantly Feeling Off or Ill

- never feeling great
- lots of bad days
- seemed to be ill constantly
- constant colds or other viral illnesses
- never felt like I recovered fully from infections

Feeling Cold

- shivering
- needing warmer clothes than others
- hands always cold
- feet constantly cold
- cold feet even with socks on
- was needing heavier covers at night

Thyroid Nodules

- some with symptoms
- some without symptoms
- throat swelling
- throat tightness

Excess Adrenaline

- felt hyper all over
- mind was going a million directions
- anxiety
- panicky
- couldn't relax
- felt shaky
- felt fearful about things

Heart (from excess adrenaline)

- rapid heart rate
- racing heart
- low heart rate
- palpitations
- heart seemed irregular
- skipped beats
- pounding heart

Hands

- loss of feeling/numbness
- shaky
- drier than I had ever had before
- nails were breaking easily
- fingers were cold
- hands were always cold

Emotional Symptoms

- feeling impatient
- irritable / on edge a lot
- felt uneasy often
- felt overwhelmed at work

- cried all the time
- mood swings
- depression that I'd never had before
- moody

Achiness
- achy back
- arms were achy
- legs felt achy

Pain
- joints
- knees
- legs
- feet
- arms
- elbows
- fingers
- palms
- groin/vaginal area
- carpal tunnel
- thyroid pain

Digestive
- delayed feeling of hunger after eating
- had to go a long time between meals before feeling hunger
- poor appetite
- stomach never feeling right
- intestines feel gaseous
- constipation
- hard little stools

Menstrual or Female Hormones

- heavy bleeding
- leakage from my breasts which made no sense
- couldn't get pregnant
- sudden long menstrual periods
- periods coming frequently
- PCOS diagnosis

Swelling

- neck became bigger
- puffy face
- puffy eye lids
- enlarged tongue
- hands
- wrists
- ankles

Skin

- flaking dandruff
- terribly dry skin
- vitiligo/whiter spots on my skin
- acne
- itchiness

Inflammation

- labs were showing it and had no idea why
- could feel inflammation in my body

Head and Neck

- migraines (worsening or new onset)
- headaches that I'd never had before
- lightheaded

- dizzy
- passing out (many mentioned teenage years, but not all)
- sore throats
- hard time swallowing
- turtlenecks were now uncomfortable
- tinnitus (ringing in the ears)

Body
- cold intolerance
- cold in my arms and legs
- low body temperature
- muscles wasting away
- weakness
- fever
- dizzy/vertigo
- numbness in hands, arms, legs or feet
- hives
- feeling hyper all over
- high blood pressure
- aches and pains in various places

Thyroid
- nodules
- felt tight on my neck
- goiter
- pain

Adrenals
- found myself with low cortisol
- anxiety
- wanted to avoid people

- felt defensive all the time
- wasn't coping well with my children
- woke up feeling bad
- bedtime insomnia
- waking up all night long

Blood Sugar Issues

- dropping blood sugar (hypoglycemia)
- blood sugar was high

Elimination Problems

- constipation (most common)
- small round stools (related to constipation)
- stopped seeing daily bowel movements
- diarrhea
- my bowels/intestines felt off/upset

Nutrient testing at doctor's office

- found myself with low iron for the first time
- low vitamin D

Plus...

Swings between hypo and hyper symptoms

Frequent ER visits

**Reading Stop the Thyroid Madness gave me my first sign that
  I had a problem**

Air hunger

Ringing in my ears

Antibodies discovery at doctor's office

REAL STORIES of Hashimoto's Patients

Renee's story: I have gone to my doctor about my problems for about 2 1/2 decades/25 years. I took forever to get over upper respiratory infection. I had joint pain, rashes and hives. My stomach never felt right. I had periodic migraines, hair loss and weight gain. Doc just said I had fibromyalgia and depression. I was told to watch my carb intake, told to join the gym, was put on sex hormones as I went into early menopause. It was only when I had to go to a walk-in clinic for one of those infections that took forever to get over that I found out I have Hashimoto's. That just kills me that it went that long before I found out.

Jessica's story: Seven years ago, when I was 32, I was noticing problems that I hadn't had before. So I went to my doctor, and she basically said it was all about getting older. ?? But then found out my TSH was in the 30's, so I was put on Synthroid. Thankfully I knew enough to say I wanted Natural Desiccated Thyroid (NDT) thanks to STTM (stopthethyroidmadness.com). She said no. She also tested my antibodies, which both were high. Yet in spite of those high levels, her explanation was that I'm just hypo. It took four more years for me to understand the significance of Hashimoto's. I changed my diet plus I got on NDT.

B.D.'s story: I've only had my TSH tested for a good 18 years, always said I'm fine. Wish I had known sooner that the TSH is stupid. Then was given a prescription of Prozac for my depression. But I always said something is not right with me! I had bouts of diarrhea, bloating and my neck always looked larger than it used to. It took me ordering my own labs to find out I had Hashimoto's plus low free T3 and low free T4. I'm now treating my antibodies with Low

Dose Naltrexone and selenium, and learning how to eat differently. I'm also now on desiccated thyroid.

Karen's story: No kidding, but I've counted seven doctors in eight years who have failed to diagnose me with Hashimoto's. It took going to a functional medicine doctor about an hour away before I finally got the real diagnosis of Hashi's. I'm working on it now and look forward to what your book will explain.

Steph's story: I am an RN and I've worked most of my career in two hospitals. It was 2008 when my antibodies were discovered, but I was told to just wait it out as there wasn't much to be done. It's wasn't fun working when you have anxiety, depression and feel awful. I felt like I should be the one in the bed. I have used Celexa to treat both my depression and panicky feelings. In 2012, I finally got the diagnosis of hypothyroidism (wonder how long I've had that). And now my antibodies were much higher. I was put on Synthroid, felt a little better. But it did nothing to control my high anxiety. Then I found out on my own that I have low cortisol. What a mess. I'm treating the low cortisol with cortisol supplementation, following Chapter 6 in the revised STTM book with my doctor, and have added T3 to my T4 with hopes of someday moving over to NDT (natural desiccated thyroid), or not, because doing both synthetics is ok. Oh and I'm using LDN (low dose naltrexone) to lower my antibodies, and I finally kicked gluten from my foods. I have hope now.

NOTES

Chapter 13

Problematic Foods as Reported by Patients

Remarkably, it appears to be quite common for certain Hashimoto's patients to have reactions to some foods. With those reactions come negative symptoms, and they make Hashimoto's worse with flares! Here is a summary of the relationship between foods and having Hashimoto's disease:

1. **With any certain food**, a large body with Hashi's may have a bad reaction, even if a small body with Hashi's will not to that certain food. Gluten is a good example for the large majority, often stated as 9 out of 10 Hashi's patients. There are other foods besides those with gluten which can cause a bad reaction.

2. **With a variety of foods,** a majority may have a bad reaction to a variety of foods, while a few may not have any bad reaction to a variety of foods.

3. The lack of obvious symptoms to certain foods may not mean there isn't a problem. For example, with the consumption of gluten, you might be someone who has no obvious negative reactions. But once you get off, you might be like some who say they do feel better.

Gluten sensitivity
vs celiac disease
vs wheat allergy

It turns out that gluten consumption is extremely problematic for most Hashimoto's patients. Not only can it promote leaky gut, but gluten can cause chronic and thus dangerous inflammation. And unfortunately, the structure of gluten molecules resembles human tissue in the eye of your mixed-up immune system. So, in those with autoimmune tendencies, antibodies will go up due to this confusion—a perfect example of cross-reactivity!

Let's dig into the different versions of gluten problems:

1. Gluten Sensitivity, also termed Non-Celiac Gluten Sensitivity (NCGS)

Not only can NCGS happen to non-Hashimoto's patients, it's certainly a common form of a gluten problem for Hashimoto's patients. It may be classified as "less severe" than the overreactive autoimmune Celiac disease, but patients who experience the bad reactions to gluten wouldn't call their symptoms "less severe".

It was originally described in the 1980's. Then in 2001, an international consensus on NCGS defined it as a *"non-allergic and non-autoimmune condition in which the consumption of gluten can lead to symptoms similar to those seen in CD.*[212]*"* As with Hashimoto's, it is far more common with women.

---

[212] https://www.ncbi.nlm.nih.gov/pmc/articles/PMC5677194/

Studies show that NCGS can trigger dysbiosis (gut bacteria imbalance) on top of the chronic and insidious inflammation it will drive. It might even make one more likely to have cognitive problems leading to dementia[213], thus the importance of getting off gluten.

Symptoms of NCGS are not only about chronic and serious inflammation, but in some, can also include bloating, diarrhea, brain fog, joint pain, numbness, depression, low iron, or abdominal pain.

A ferritin test can reveal the inflammation i.e. if the result is close to 100 or higher in women, or higher than the 120's in men. Ferritin is measuring storage iron, and the body tends to push iron into storage in the presence of inflammation to stop the iron from feeding the inflammation.

If ferritin doesn't reveal one's inflammation, the other tests are CRP (C-reactive protein) or ESR (erythrocyte sedimentation rate). Damaging inflammation was strongly manifested in a dear friend of mine with NCGS if she continually failed to get off gluten.

The problem with the inflammation caused by NCFS is that it's a trigger towards worsening Hashimoto's. Removing gluten-containing foods can lower antibodies and reverse the bad symptoms in the majority, as reported by patients with a commitment to removing gluten from their consumption.

Non-Celiac Gluten Sensitivity can show anti-gliadin antibodies (AGAs) of IgG class rather than the Tissue Transglutaminase Antibodies (tTG-IgA) that the majority of Celiac disease patients will show. AGAs are anti-food protein antibodies, not related to autoimmune issues, and will disappear after 6 months of going gluten-free.

---

[213] https://www.ncbi.nlm.nih.gov/pubmed/29247390

2. Celiac Disease

This severe form of a gluten reaction is a problematic autoimmune condition like Hashimoto's, but the overreactive immune system attacks transglutaminase within the intestines. Transglutaminase is a naturally occurring binding enzyme (also known as "meat glue" since it's used by the meat industry to bond meats together). It can be found in imitation crab, certain fish balls, and even in some hams, thus why it's important to find out where it is.

Studies show that gut dysbiosis (bacteria imbalance) is a significant factor with Celiac, but it's not clear if Celiac causes dysbiosis or the other way around. The role of gut dysbiosis has even been emphasized with NCGS (#1).

The attack caused by Celiac in the intestines triggers a reaction which can cause damage to the villi, tiny fingerlike projections that line the small intestine.[214] These villi are how you absorb nutrients from your intestines, so they are quite important.

Celiac tends to run in families. The immunity-related gene called HLA-DQ may be a strong cause, but it may have a partner in crime— environmental triggers like infections, toxins, even the addition of transglutaminase in foods.

The risk of acquiring Celiac when you already have Hashimoto's is high, possibly since they both share some of the same gene mutations. But it's environmental factors with the genes that may push someone over the edge.

Besides inflammation, symptoms can include bloating, joint pain, diarrhea, hair loss, weight loss, fatigue, fertility problems and more.

The Celiac Disease Foundation states the most accurate test is the **Tissue Transglutaminase Antibodies (tTG-IgA)** while consuming

---

[214] https://www.archivesofpathology.org/doi/pdf/10.5858/arpa.2012-0354-OA

gluten. Ask your doctor about this test. For the very small percentage that the latter test might miss, there are other tests:

IgA Endomysial antibody (EMA)
Total serum IgA
Deaminated gliadin peptide (DGP IgA and IgG)

One good news about Celiac and the damaged villi: once a patient gets off gluten, the villi can heal over time. But it can take up to a few years of being consistently off gluten.

3. Wheat Allergy

In a wheat allergy, you will react to any of hundreds of proteins within wheat, of which gluten is only one of those proteins. Wheat allergies can be identified by IgE antibodies (as compared to IgA with Celiac) and which can produce a fairly sudden response in your body, or a slightly delayed response. Symptoms from released chemicals can include itching, hives, swelling lips or tongue, rashes, nausea and even nasal congestion.

Those with wheat allergies might be able to tolerate gluten in non-wheat products. If an adult, wheat allergies can be a lifetime reaction, so completely avoiding wheat is important.

It's recommended to consult an allergist about testing if a gluten allergy is suspected. They may do a skin prick test and/or blood tests for the IgE antibodies.

A wheat allergy is mistakenly called a gluten allergy.

The antibodies mentioned above

When you see *IgA, IgD, IgE, IgG or IgM*, they all refer to immunoglobulins, which is another name for antibodies produced by your immune system to battle any unwanted substance. Even a healthy immune system makes antibodies in response to foreign substances like bacteria, viruses or fungus like candida. They can also be produced in response to pollen, dust in the air, pet hair, and foods.

But with problematic autoimmune overreactions, your body produces way too many antibodies. It's overkill! Thus, they can spread to your healthy tissue.

I define each of the antibodies at the end of Chapter 1.

List of Problematic Foods as Reported by Hashimoto's Patients

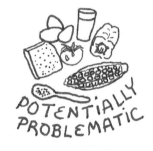

Below, from the responses of over 400 Hashimoto's patients over the years, I list…

• the foods mentioned by Hashimoto's patients as causing reactions

• what the noted reactions were based on consuming these foods.

Some patients listed a single symptom; most listed multiple symptoms. Check what you identify with below, and even write in your own.

GRAINS/WHEAT

- hives
- itchiness (ears)
- water retention in my tissues
- swelling (face, eyelids, body, etc.)
- red face/warm
- neck and upper chest turn red
- tired/fatigued
- angry feelings
- headache
- under eye dark circles

- nose dripping
- bloating
- burping
- diarrhea
- constipation
- achy
- brain fog
- inflammation
- gas
- knee pain
- other pains
- rising antibodies
- nausea
- the sweats
- stomach pain
- indigestion
- stomach grumbling
- feel sick
- extremely hungry
- grumpy
- less energy

DAIRY (another common reactive food for Hashi's patients)

- digestive problems
- hives
- rashes
- rough skin in places
- diarrhea
- asthma

- throat mucus
- sinus problems
- indigestion
- rising antibodies
- swelling
- pain
- coughing and acid reflux

SUGAR

- feelings of panic
- rising antibodies
- bloating
- see spots
- dizziness

NIGHTSHADES (Tomatoes, potatoes, eggplant, bell peppers, paprika, etc.)

- achy joints
- diarrhea
- vomiting
- acid reflux
- headaches

CORN

- made me feel off
- rashes
- indigestion

SOY

- headache and dizziness
- bloating
- feel bad
- face swelling
- hand swelling
- diarrhea
- fatigue
- sleep problems

EGGS

- stuffy nose
- headache
- feel bad
- gas
- stomach pain

SEAFOOD (may be more about an allergy)

- feel off
- hives
- swelling

CASHEWS

- hives
- feel off
- breathing issue

ALCOHOL

- headache the next morning
- joint pain
- fast heart rate
- red face/warm

CHOCOLATE (may be a reaction to milk products)

- feel bad
- hives

BANANAS

- mouth tingles
- rash
- burning stomach

BEANS

- excess gas

GOITROGENS like raw broccoli, brussel sprouts, cabbage

- gas
- bloating
- stomach pain

CAFFEINE in foods or drinks

- muscle spasms
- migraines
- anxiety
- irregular heartbeats
- chest tightening

HIGH OXALATE FOODS (spinach, tea, dark chocolate, etc.)

- vaginal pain
- feel bad
- burning urine

PORK

- diarrhea
- gut pain
- stomach gurgling
- GI tract problems

BEEF

- flu-like symptoms
- digestive problems
- diarrhea or gas

Will you react in any of the stated ways that others react? Some will; some won't. Or you will react to a food not even listed here. It's simply very individual what will trigger symptoms, and what won't.

There are even a few individuals with years of having Hashi's, yet who react to none of the foods. The individual differences are there, even if majority can react to certain foods.

It's clearly very important to find out WHY you react to these foods, because if it's Celiac disease, it can create lifelong damage. Even inflammation caused by a sensitivity (#1) or an allergy (#3) can cause you a host of problems, as uncontrolled inflammation can spread to different parts of your body, plus make your antibodies worse.

Ingredient terms that can mean gluten

- *Barley grass or enzymes (can be cross contaminated)*
- *Bulgur (a form of wheat)*
- *Couscous (made from wheat)*
- *Dextrin (by itself or in a longer word—can be from wheat)*
- *Farina (made from wheat)*
- *Hordeum*
- *Malt (made from barley)*
- *Seitan (made from wheat gluten; often in vegetarian meals)*
- *Semolina*
- *Spelt (type of wheat also known as farro or dinkel)*
- *Vegetable protein (can come from wheat)*
- *Wheat germ oil or extract (can be contaminated)*
- *Yeast extract (may come from barley)*

Here are 9 recommended solutions reported by Hashi's patients or experts

1) Remove offending food from your diet.
2) Research if an offending food might be hidden in other foods.
3) With gluten, pay attention to gluten food residues on your cutting board, knives or other utensils, racks in oven, etc.

4) If unsure which foods are causing problems, Hashi's patients are recommending an elimination diet, i.e. stop eating some of the most common problematic foods like grains (gluten), all dairy, soy of any kind, eggs, sugar and corn for up to 3 weeks. Then introduce one food at a time, eating twice a day. After a few days, notice any return of any negative symptom(s). It might help to write down the symptoms—the above list will help identify possible signs. NOTE: this may not be a good idea if there are serious allergy issues to certain foods.

5) Talk to your doctor about reliable tests.

6) Read about Leaky Gut in Chapter 10 and how to treat it.

7) Rotate your good tolerable foods to spread the nutrients around.

8) Eat more raw foods which you tolerate for added nutritional benefit and micronutrients.

9) Consider particular diet protocols—see below.

Diet Protocols to Consider as Recommended by Patients

How to eat??

Below are four ways of eating, often mentioned by various Hashi's patients, which are stated as making a big difference in lowering antibodies, curtailing inflammation, healing the gut and/or feeling much better again. See which makes sense for YOU. There are numerous websites to read on each of the diets listed.

About the terms Keto or Ketogenic: When you see reference to these words , they refer to a diet being very low carb and substantially higher in fat. Your liver will convert the consumed fat into fatty acids, then to the molecules called ketones. Ketones (acetoacetate, beta-hydroxybutyrate, and then acetone) are used as fuel when carbs are low and less available. Not everyone tolerates carbs that low.

IMPORTANT TO NOTE: if any diet causes you to feel low energy or tired, you probably need more healthy carbs incorporated into the diet.

GAPS diet: GAPS stands for Gut and Psychology Syndrome and is considered a keto way of eating. It was originally based on the Specific Carbohydrate Diet (SCD) created by Dr. Sidney Valentine, and then adjusted by Natasha Campbell-McBride, MD. The GAPS diet will remove foods that can be damaging to the gut like grains, starches, and sugars, and subbing very nutrient-dense foods to promote gut healing. There are six stages of this diet. Check out *https://www. gapsdiet.com /*

Autoimmune Paleo (AIP) diet: This extremely strict diet removes gut-irritating foods, thus can lower antibodies and the inflammation caused by them. It can be ideal for those who have a serious autoimmune problem and leaky gut. The foods eliminated are all grains, legumes, dairy, nuts, seeds, eggs, nightshades, most liquid oils, alcohol, NSAIDs (non-steroidal anti-inflammatory drugs like aspirin and ibuprofen), sugar, starches, fruits, yeast and most all processed foods. After being on this diet for up to 60 days, patients report reintroducing one food at a time to see if there is still a reaction, or not. The standard AIP diet is not considered a strict keto way of eating, but one can use keto low carb recipes to make AIP more keto. Check out www.thepaleomom.com/start-here/the-autoimmune-pro-tocol/   And here's another good one: *https://unboundwellness.com/*

Paleo Diet: This is less strict than the autoimmune paleo and based on foods that "Paleolithic cavemen" might have gathered and eaten, which includes lean meats, fish, fruits, vegetables, nuts and seeds. It limits dairy, legumes and grains. It's not unusual for those who used the strict AIP diet successfully to then move to the paleo diet. Check out: *http://paleodiet.com/* There are also many great books on the Paleo diet, such as *The Paleo Thyroid Solution: Stop Feeling Fat, Foggy, And Fatigued At The Hands Of Uninformed Doctors - Reclaim Your Health!* by Elle Russ.

Low FODMAP diet: This is a diet low in fermentable carbs, since the latter can aggravate gut symptoms in sensitive individuals, especially with irritable bowel syndrome. FODMAP stands for this mouthful: fermentable oligo- di- mono-saccharides and polyols. The latter include the following foods which this diet will stay very low:

- Oligo-saccharides: Grains like wheat and rye, certain fruits and veggies, onions and garlic, plus legumes.
- Di-saccharides: This includes lactose products like milk, soft chee-ses and yogurt.
- Mono-saccharides: This is about fructose fruits like figs and man-goes, sweeteners like honey and agave.
- Polyols: sorbitol and mannitol which can occur in different fruit and veggies.

Check it out here: https://www.monashfodmap.com/

TIDBITS

- There are some pretty odd things that can contain gluten, thus the importance of reading ingredients. They are: PlayDoh, some hotdogs, certain lipsticks or balms, some lotions, some moisturizers, and malt vinegar in pickles.

- Have a gluten problem? Be careful of ice cream with cookies or brownies mixed in!

NOTES

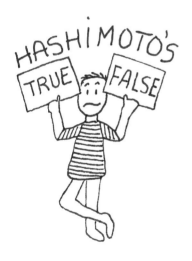

Chapter 14   Hashimoto's Whoppers

No, I'm not talking about an American fast food hamburger. :) This is about falsehoods, exaggerations or myths, aka "whoppers" in opinions or suppositions.

And unfortunately, there have occurred an awful lot of whoppers over the years about Hashimoto's disease, whether from our doctors or each other, and which our experiences and wisdom prove to be quite wrong. Let's go over several of them:

Whopper #1:

"All you need to test is one thyroid antibody to reveal Hashimoto's."

There are two main thyroid antibodies pertaining to Hashimoto's: anti-thyroid peroxidase (anti-TPO) and anti-thyroglobulin (anti-Tg). Research shows that the anti-TPO will show up in the highest percentage of Hashimoto's cases, up to 90% depending on who you read. So perhaps because of that, your doctor may think it's just fine to only test anti-TPO.

Yet, years of observations have revealed that some Hashi's patients only have a high anti-Tg with a perfectly low, in-range, anti-TPO. It's stated that up to 80% have this one. But that's still a high amount. Thus, if the doctor only does the anti-TPO, the diagnosis might be "No Hashimoto's", when in fact, you have it.

Whopper #2:

"You just need to let your Hashimoto's run its course."

How often we have heard this clueless pronouncement from doctors to so many thyroid patients. And bottom line, it means to continue having the miseries of the attack for years. No way. There are great strategies to lower the attack, if not totally stop it, as you'll see in Chapters 16 and 17.

Whopper #3:

"All Hashi's patients should *completely avoid* iodine supplements." (or any other negative leaning, anti-iodine comment)

Any negative-leaning statement against iodine fails to note that there are a body of Hashi's patients reporting that their careful use of iodine was the sole reason their antibodies came down! That is huge. Others report obvious benefits. So no, it's a whopper. And too many Hashi's patients have found their iodine levels too low.

Now granted, some Hashi's patients see their antibodies go up when starting iodine. That can be due to the stress of the iodine-induced toxin release of halides like bromide, chloride, and fluoride. So, the answer, say experts, is to prepare with companion nutrients (coined by Lynne Farrow, author of The Iodine Crisis). They can include selenium, magnesium, vitamin C, B2 and B3, plus sodium. And for other Hashi's patients, that can be about going up slow and staying low in the final amount, yet still getting the benefits.

Bottom line, do your research and see what you think is right for you! But don't get caught up in the excessive negative-leaning opinions against iodine for "all". This is not talking about too-high amounts.

Whopper #4:

"Goitrogens like soy, broccoli, cauliflower, collard greens, kale, etc. should be *completely avoided* by Hashi's patients."

The trip-up in this whopper is the part of the phrase that states "should be completely avoided". That hasn't been true for most patients. Sure, whether with Hashi's or non-Hashi's hypothyroidism, "excess" goitrogen intake has been implicated in making you susceptible to having a goiter, or enlargement of your thyroid, or reduced thyroid function. Goitrogens are known to interfere with iodine uptake in the thyroid gland, thus interfere with sufficient levels of thyroid hormones T3 and T4.

So, what's the safest way to eat goitrogens? First, not every day.

Spreading out one's consumption is usually fine. And second, if you boil them, you will be removing approximately 90% of the goitrogens.

Check out a list of goitrogens here: https://stopthethyroidmadness. com/goitrogens/

Whopper #5:

"If there is no one observed in my family or ancestry with autoimmune diseases, I won't have it either."

Granted, having a family history of autoimmune diseases seems to increase the risk of you acquiring an autoimmune disease, as well. But there are also individuals with Hashimoto's who find no instance of autoimmune diseases in their family or recent ancestors (or they don't recognize autoimmune diseases).

Whopper #6:

"All I need to do is 'eat healthy' as a Hashimoto's patient."

The problem is that recommended "healthy food" lists can include certain dairy products, nuts, and seeds, nightshade vegetables like tomatoes and bell peppers, and high fiber breads—any of which can raise one's antibodies and inflammation in sensitive individuals. So "healthy" doesn't always equal "appropriate" if you have an autoimmune disease like Hashi's.

Whopper #7:

"Hashimoto's patients should absolutely not use natural desiccated thyroid (NDT) since it's like throwing fire on one's antibodies."

There are a large and growing body of Hashi's patient who have soared on NDT for years now. In fact, there are some who have reported that it was their NDT alone which lowered their antibodies (similar to those whose iodine use did the same).

Now it's true that at first, NDT can cause one's antibodies to rise. Thyroid hormones are the enemy! But a large body of Hashi's patients stated that the rise of antibodies ended once they got optimal on NDT (a free T3 towards the top part of the range with a mid-range free T4). Others used a medication like Low Dose Naltrexone to get stubborn antibodies down, or other strategies, while feeling the benefit with NDT for their now hypothyroid state. LDN is mentioned in Chapter 16.

Whopper #8:

"Endocrinologists are the best doctors for me."

Though there can be exceptions, Endocrinologists as a whole have been reported by patients as being T4-only obsessed (Synthroid, levothyroxine, Eltroxin, Oroxine, and etc.), plus have an obsession with the worst test ever invented—the TSH lab test.

So too often, Endo's have been reported as the worst doctors for Hashimoto's patients. Instead, patients report having a better chance with "Functional Medicine" doctors, seeking those who will listen to their own intelligence and wisdom. No matter who you find, be prepared that YOU will have teach them (if they will listen).

Whopper #9:

"With Hashimoto's, I need to have my thyroid removed".

In the vast majority of cases, there was and is no need to have the thyroid removed, lament Hashi's patients who did. Instead, there are many good strategies to reverse symptoms caused by the autoimmune attack on the thyroid. The exception: if an enlarged thyroid is causing problems breathing or eating. Or if one also has thyroid cancer.

Whopper #10:

"I am now healed because of what I eat."

For Hashimoto's patients, it is key in one's treatment of Hashi's to be aware of inflammation triggering foods and avoiding them. The more common ones expressed by patients are: most grains, dairy, certain nightshades, sugar, eggs, gluten-containing foods, and corn.

But though avoiding triggering foods is highly important to put the Hashi's attack into remission, it doesn't mean your "thyroid" itself is healed. Damage may have already occurred and that can be evident by the free T3 and free T4. If they are below mid-range, that represents a damaged thyroid. So thyroid medication like Natural Desiccated Thyroid, or using both synthetic T4 and T3, plus finding one's optimal dose, are needed.

Whopper #11:

"I will be fine by just cutting down on gluten."

The problem is the "cutting down", which may not be enough. Consuming gluten is a huge trigger for rising antibodies in 9 out of 10 Hashi's patients. But cutting down has proven to not be enough for the majority. For some, even tiny hidden amounts have caused problems, as well as cross-contamination in other foods.

Whopper #12:

"I did the two antibodies tests and they were fine, so I don't have Hashimoto's."

There are a small body of Hashi's patients with negative or in-range antibody results, yet they are noticing a swelling where their thyroid is, or other symptoms of a failing thyroid gland. It's called Seronegative Hashimoto's, or seronegative autoimmune thyroiditis. Another potential clue are the antibodies tests showing a result at the top of the range, even if still in-range. The final and most conclusive test is an ultrasound to look at the appearance of your thyroid. It will have a hypoechoic pattern, meaning darker areas compared to other areas.

Whopper #13:

"I feel fine on Synthroid/Levothyroxine/Eltroxin/Oroxine— all T4-only medications. We're all different."

While it's true that at first, some Hashi's patients do feel fine with T4-only meds, years of reports reveal that sooner or later, it backfires, as the body it not meant to live for conversion alone, i.e. from T4 to the active T3. A healthy thyroid gives some direct T3!

And with Hashimoto's patients, if inflammation is still a problem, that T4 is going to convert to rising amounts of reverse T3 (RT3) in the presence of inflammation. The more RT3 we convert to, the less T3 will get to the cells.

Giving ourselves all five hormones (as Natural Desiccated Thyroid does) or adding T3 to T4, or even being just T3 (multi-dosed) has proven to be a far better treatment. Being optimal is important, too, along with the right amount of iron and cortisol.

Whopper #14:

"I did terrible on Natural Desiccated Thyroid NDT (or T3), thus it's not for me."

From years of reports and experiences, Stop the Thyroid Madness reports two key reasons why someone may have problems, and they are correctible...

1. Staying on too low a dose.

This happens when your doctor holds you hostage to the TSH lab test, or simply keeps you too low due to lack of knowledge or fear. As a result, the adrenals become alarmed, releasing excess adrenaline. Patient reports reveal that the solution is to raise NDT until optimal, which can mean teaching your doctor or finding a much better one. Optimal for most puts the free T3 towards the top part of the range and the free T4 midrange. Both, say patients. It will also put the TSH below range, which that is not the same as Graves' disease. Nor does the low TSH from being optimal on NDT equal bone loss or heart problems, as too many doctors will falsely proclaim. But now read #2 below....

2. Raising in the presence of inadequate iron or problematic cortisol levels.

You are destined to have reactions if you are raising NDT or T3 in the presence of non-optimal iron levels, or high or low cortisol. Symptoms of inadequate iron include rising RT3 and worsening of hypothyroid symptoms. Symptoms of a cortisol problem range from rising RT3 (due to high cortisol) to palpitations, fast heartrate, anxiety and more (due to low cortisol.) See Chapter 11, and for more details, and read *https://stopthethyroidmadness.com/iron-and-cortisol*

Whopper #15:

"Epstein Barr Virus is the sole reason to have Hashimoto's."

Epstein Barr Virus (EBV) is a member of the Herpes virus family. It's the very same virus that causes Mononucleosis, aka "mono" or the kissing disease. And whether we had mono or not, literature states that anywhere around 95% of adults have this virus laying dormant in their bodies. So in the presence of any kind of chronic stress, this dormant virus can reactivate. And a reactivated EBV can trigger anti-thyroid antibodies. But though we know that an active EBV virus can be a Hashi's trigger, research and common sense concludes it's *not* the only contributory factor for autoimmune thyroiditis.

NOTES

40 Most Frustrating Aspects of Having Hashimoto's disease: From the Words of Patients Worldwide

The following countdown represents what most frustrates Hashimoto's patients over the years, in no special order.

Which do you identify with?

40. The constant back and forth in my health / never knowing what will hit next, what will cause my Hashi's to flare, how I will flare.

39. Puffy eyelids, under eyes, face, anywhere on my body

38. Sleep issues (insomnia, waking up often, feeling unrefreshed when waking up in the morning)

37. Not knowing if symptoms are the Hashi's or Lyme or other problems I have

36. Food intolerances; can't eat foods I used to love

35. Lack of libido / frustrated partner

34. My changing moods

33. Losing friends because I can't do things

32. Having to cancel plans due to my problems

31. Constipation; diarrhea

30. Fatigue!! (ever-ending, severe, chronic, debilitating, life-sucking)

29. Weight gain / difficulty losing (missing clothes I used to fit in)

28. Fertility / miscarriage issues

27. Just having it

26. Feeling cold all the time

25. Brain fog

24. Having other autoimmune issues with it

23. Hair loss

22. All the years before finding out what was wrong

21. Wiping out after activity / having to constantly calculate if I can do this or that without crashing

20. Depression

19. Swings between hyper and hypo

18. Anxiety

17. Loss of my former self

16. Family or friends not understanding a thing, aka "But you don't look sick."

15. Having to explain why I can't eat gluten

14. When good medications change

13. Stupidly thinking that doctors would help me, so I didn't need to get informed

12. Achy joints / pain / muscle weakness

11. Dry skin

10. My reactions to foods

9. Less able to cope with normal stresses

8. Finding myself with low iron

7. Realizing I shouldn't have had my thyroid removed (exception is cancer)

6. The heart palpitations, fast heartrate, irregular beats

5. Eating out and the challenges it presents because of food reactions

4. Getting sicker easier than I used to

3. Controlling the inflammation

2. Having to be my own advocate when I need help

AND THE NUMBER ONE, MOST OFTEN MENTIONED FRUSTRATION....

1. Doctors

Here are actual comments made by numerous Hashimoto's patients over the years about their doctor or doctors.

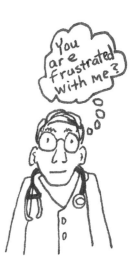

- doesn't listen
- knows so little about Hashi's
- told me to let it run its course
- told me there's nothing to do
- showed little empathy / cold demeanor
- doesn't understand triggers
- thinks typing on her computer is all she needs to do when I'm there
- pushes T4 meds
- has little knowledge about Natural Desiccated Thyroid (NDT) or T3
- let me be on NDT, but kept me too low and refused to raise
- only goes by the TSH
- has limited / backwards knowledge about adrenal issues
- dismisses me

- refuses to believe I might have my own wisdom
- left me undiagnosed for years/decades
- said my symptoms were due to something else
- dismisses good information I've gotten from Stop the Thyroid Madness
- dismisses my own knowledge
- told me to ignore what's on the internet
- has no clue how to read lab work
- everything is normal, normal
- my doc told me I'd get a heart attack on NDT (natural desiccated thyroid)
- told me my weight gain means I'm eating too much
- said I needed to exercise more—really??
- very, very frustrated with the medical system
- diagnosed with fibromyalgia instead of understanding Hashi's and the correct way to treat
- going to multiple doctors who end up knowing nothing
- thinks Synthroid is the way to go
- doesn't believe me when I describe what's going on
- having to battle doctors
- doctors who think their medical school degrees on the wall equals being knowledgeable
- said I'm not suitable for T3 when I clearly need it
- he looked at me like I was a hypochondriac
- not being heard
- having to spend money for terrible doctors
- my doctor gaslighting me, saying it's not as I see it
- just finding a doctor to do the right tests, understand the results, give the right meds
- told me I'm tired because I'm a mother
- not believing me when I said that Levothyroxine is not working

for me.

- doctors who say you can't blame everything on my thyroid problem
- the burden of having to teach your doctor, yet having to pay him
- dealing with lousy Endocrinologists
- each doctor as bad as the last one
- have lost faith in all doctors—they are inept
- doctors who treat you like you are the bad guy for having knowledge opposite his or her own
- arrogance
- told me I needed counseling rather than understanding hypothyroid, brain, and depression
- treated me like I had a mental health disorder
- having to diagnose myself
- the headache of finding a better doctor

Yes, a large body of patients express high frustration about their doctors. And I suspect that the majority of patients reading this will identify with many of the above. Granted, some Hashi's patients are lucky and have found a doctor who gets it about better treatment. But it takes work. And there appear to be far too many doctors who don't get it. Thus, the importance of this book, as there are many steps you can do yourself with your diet supplements, moderating stress and more.

How to find a much better doctor

As far as trying to find a much better doctor...a good first idea is asking other Hashi's patients if they found a good doctor. And if they say yes, ask what makes their doctor a good doctor. You are looking for a doctor you can teach, honestly, which this book will help you to do, as well the Stop the Thyroid Madness website and books.

Another fruitful way to find a potentially better doctor? Start calling pharmacies and ask which doctors are prescribing NDT (natural desiccated thyroid) or T3. It's at least a start.

Informed patients will tell you that it helps to find one who is open-minded about using better thyroid medications than Synthroid or Levothyroxine—a body is not meant to live for conversion alone, i.e. T4 to T3, the active thyroid hormone. Too many issues can inhibit that conversion, sadly, sooner or later. Even a healthy thyroid gives us direct T3 instead of just conversion.

And the cherry on top is if you can convince a doctor to stop using the TSH as a measure of whether you are on enough of Natural Desiccated Thyroid (NDT) or T3. When optimal, the TSH will naturally fall below range with no problems. To the contrary, doctor, our low TSH is NOT the same as what happens with Graves' disease. It goes low because we are taking over the job of the TSH. It's far more about the free T3 and free T4 and where in the range they fall. Optimal puts the free T3 towards the top area and the free T4 midrange. Both.

Problems with NDT (natural desiccated thyroid), T4/T3, or T3: Two correctable reasons

1) **Staying on too low a dose.** Staying too low will eventually kick in excess adrenaline,, patients have noted, which causes heart palps, fast heartrate, anxiety or etc. Symptoms of our hypothyroidism usually get worse, too.

2) **Having inadequate iron and/or a cortisol problem.** Raising NDT with inadequate iron or inflammation pushes Reverse T3 (RT3) up, the inactive hormone, thus we feel more hypo. Raising NDT or T3 with a cortisol problem causes the T3 to pool, meaning going high in the blood and not making it to the cells. Raising

with a cortisol problem has also caused hyper-like symptoms like anxiety, heart palps, fast heartrate etc. This is all why having *optimal iron and cortisol* is crucial to successfully raise either natural desiccated thyroid or T3...without problems

Here's a page with patient experiences and wisdom on both the latter *https://stopthethyroidmadness.com/iron-and-cortisol* Hopefully this is a topic you can teach your doctor, as they tend to blame the meds.

Postscript: In the November 2014 magazine Atlantic, there's an insightful article titled *"Doctors Tell All—and It's Bad"* with the byline *"A crop of books by disillusioned physicians reveals a corrosive doctor-patient relationship at the heart of our health-care crisis."* A worthy read. It's also here if you care to type it all out in your phone or computer browser: *https://www. theatlantic.com/magazine/archive/2014/11/doctors-tell-all- and-its-bad/380785/* If the URL changes, just search the title on the internet.

NOTES

Chapter 16

95 Testimonies:
How Patients are Lowering their Antibodies / Heading Towards Remission

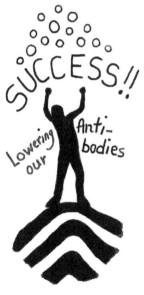

Ready?

Here are 95 Hashimoto's success strategies as expressed by real patients. The strategies represent what they are doing to lower their anti-thyroid antibodies towards remission and to prevent flares.

Are all these success strategies for you? Definitely many are, while some may not be. For example, though the biggest majority see success in lowering antibodies by avoiding gluten, a small minority didn't achieve that success. But seeing such a majority have success going gluten free makes it a very worthy mention.

Or someone may have no issue with eggs or sugar while others definitely see problems consuming either!

Or some, if they use iodine, will see iodine alone lowering their antibodies. Others may have problems and need to go low and slow towards success.

This would be a good chapter to circle or highlight those strategies that interest you, or those supplements or ideas you want to add to your own treatment protocols.

NOTE: Definitions of many words or acronyms below this list.

1. I use natural cleaners now, NDT, gluten free.

2. Iodine and Inositol to throw my antibodies into remission.

3. LDN has been my miracle in lowering antibodies.

4. Removing gluten mostly, cutting down on dairy to be totally off. Eventually sugar.

5. LDN has been my miracle in bringing my antibodies down.

6. I use NDT in optimal levels to lower antibodies, plus do yoga.

7. Black Cumin Seed Oil because of reading it may repair damaged thyroid tissue; also gluten free

8. I have done the Autoimmune Protocol way of eating and it totally brought my antibodies down. I now follow just the Paleo way of eating as a maintenance.

9. LDN (low dose naltrexone), cutting way down on sugar, and going totally gluten free have lowered my antibodies.

10. With Lugols iodine, my Tgab went from 214 down to 62 so far. I'm still working on my TPOab with selenium.

11. I have gone to keto way of eating and my antibodies are down.

12. My focus in on eating healthier. I eat berries, non-dairy yogurt, lots of veggies, bone broth.

13. I have removed all dairy, all gluten and cutting down carbs.

14. I have eliminated the foods that cause me problems by symptoms, take selenium and iodine, and my antibodies are going down.

15. Low carb and grain free. Antibodies fell.

16. LDN

17. I have done gluten and dairy free.

18. I now eat Paleo and am walking more to help keep inflammation in check.

19. Strictly Keto and so far, my antibodies are down below 1000 and I expect to see them further down soon.

20. Inositol

21. I am using selenium 400 mcg and eating healthier, so I have brought my anti-TPO down from 822 down to 198 in several months.

22. I am gluten free, dairy free, soy free and my antibodies are going down.

23. I do Keto and have been in remission for two years.

24. I am avoiding soy, gluten, dairy and processed foods. I also take minerals, omega 3, vitamin D and am feeling so much better.

25. I use selenium to lower my high anti-TPO and it's working.

26. I am one of those who lowered my antibodies just with Natural Desiccated Thyroid.

27. Gluten free, soy free, exercise.

28. AIP has been the main way I've lowered my antibodies.

29. AIP, desiccated thyroid and selenium

30. AIP way of eating has lowered my antibodies

31. Compounded T3 has alone brought my high antibodies substantially down.

32. I am using selenium, 5% iodine and vitamin A

33. LDN, AIP and NDT.

34. LDN has been the biggest help, plus going gluten free.

35. Being gluten free has made the biggest difference in lowering my antibodies. Also dairy, sugar and eggs.

36. LDN has lowered my antibodies.

37. Wobenzym supplement and selenium.

38. Removed both gluten and sugar

39. Have gone gluten free and treating my gut

40. LDN

41. In over a year, turmeric alone brought my antibodies down from 577 to 85.

42. Totally gluten free and keto

43. Keto

44. AIP

45. I have removed foods I am allergic to (via testing is how I found out). Antibodies are down!

46. Keto with NDT have lowered my antibodies.

47. LDN and I cut down on dairy and gluten. Big difference.

48. Low Dose Naltrexone (LDN), compounded, plus selenium and eating clean

49. Going off dairy

50. Eliminating sugar

51. No sugar and LDN.

52. I am doing the AIP diet with LDN—seeing antibodies lower

53. LDN with selenium, no gluten, dairy or soy

54. I went gluten free, then removed all milk products so far, and my antibodies have gone down 700 points.

55. Turmeric for my inflammation and selenium to lower my TPO antibodies. So far, down by half.

56. NDT alone lowered my antibodies

57. T3 and iodine

58. Have cut down sugar, selenium, herbs. Antibodies down.

59. I am doing a whole food diet, plus I'm gluten free

60. Ketogenic

61. Selenium alone lowered my antibodies

62. I am now sleeping 8 hours no matter what; Keto and removed dairy.

63. Betaine to treat my low stomach acid, plus I use NAC for glutathione, and am gluten free.

64. I use vitamin D, 200 mg selenium, all the B's, NAC, and liver support.

65. Avoiding stress and gluten free.

66. NDT, selenium, gluten free

67. NDT and gluten free.

68. Iodine. Antibodies down.

69. Treating inflammation (fish oil, curcumin), iodine. (Don't listen to iodine nay-sayers. It works.)

70. Gluten avoider, using Curcumin and antibodies down

71. NAC and gluten free

72. Gluten free!!

73. Autoimmune diet and lowering stress has helped.

74. Gluten free.

75. Gluten & dairy free.

76. LDN has lowered my antibodies.

77. Gluten free was like a miracle

78. NAC, inositol to lower mine. Work in progress.

79. Selenium

80. Inositol and looking at transfer factors

81. Free of gluten, dairy and eggs.

82. LDN

83. Removing toxins like my breast implants

84. Iodine, NDT, minerals, NAC, liver detox, gluten and sugar free.

85. Iodine, gluten and dairy free-no more stomach issues.

86. Gluten free, dairy free, using vitamin D supp, LDN

87. Totally gluten free plus LDN

88. NP Thyroid and optimal.

89. Free of dairy, caffeine, gluten, soy

90. AIP

91. No more alcohol, NAC, no gluten, dairy, eggs, soy

92. LDN—speed lightning lowering of antibodies

93. Gluten/dairy/soy/sugar free. Antibodies down a lot.

94. AIP lowered my antibodies

95. T3-only. Lower antibodies.

96. Paleo diet. Antibodies down 85 pts so far.

97. Iodine did it alone for me.

98. Finally removed all gluten and sugar. Antibodies lowered.

About Low Dose Naltrexone (LDN)

You may have noticed the mention of Low Dose Naltrexone (LDN) from several patient testimonies. Turns out it's a pretty effective treatment to cause an endorphin release which in turn evens out your immune response. The result is better control of antibodies.

Starting doses of LDN by patients can be as low as .5, then increased slowly. Some increase by .5 every week, but others feel the need to raise much slower to prevent problems. Effective doses seem to be 2-3 mg, but some patients feel they need to go up to 4.5 mg to see good results. LDN is via compounding pharmacies and in a slow-release form.

Have patience, as the good effects may take several weeks to a few months, say patient reports.

Some patients report that in the first week of LDN use, their nighttime dreams are much more vivid, and sometimes sleep is disturbed. It eventually goes away. But if your side effects are bad or last longer, the recommendation is to lower LDN for about 7 days, then make a slow move back up.[215] Moving LDN to the morning may be better for those with bad side effects, say experts.

LDN can block the effect of pain medications if you are on them, i.e. it blocks opioid receptors.

---

[215] https://www.ldnresearchtrust.org/how-naltrexone-works

What about red and near-infrared light therapy?

This treatment protocol is called photobiomodulation (PBM) and several studies imply it can help lower antibodies.[216] The question is if it's transient or not.

> ## TERMS

AIP: This stands for Autoimmune Paleo, a way of eating that can calm inflammation. It's a version of the Paleo diet but stricter. It's mostly about vegetables (not nightshades), fruits, grass fed meats/poultry, seafood, fats, healthy fermented foods, bone broth, etc.[217]

Betaine: Usually termed Betaine HCl, which stands for Betaine Hydrochloride. Since hypothyroidism will often lower stomach acid levels (gastric or hydrochloric acid), we need to increase the levels. Otherwise, Hashimoto's patients with low stomach acid become more susceptible to having low nutrients (it's why we can see iron, B12, Vitamin D fall and more), SIBO (small intestinal bacterial overgrowth), and worsening food reactions since food we eat is not being broken down well due to low stomach acid.[218]

Black Cumin Seed oil is extracted from the seeds of Nigella sativa, mostly growing in Asia. Stated to be effective against inflammation, many illnesses and even cancer.[219] Research shows it helping to reduce antibodies,[220] and so do Hashi's patient experiences.

Curcumin: A bright yellow substance called a curcuminoid which is found in turmeric (which you might even see in your own kitchen

---

[216] https://www.hindawi.com/journals/ije/2018/8387530/
[217] https://aiplifestyle.com/what-is-autoimmune-protocol-diet/
[218] http://stopthethyroidmadness.com/stomach-acid
[219] https://www.ncbi.nlm.nih.gov/pmc/articles/PMC3252704/
[220] https://www.ncbi.nlm.nih.gov/pmc/articles/PMC5112739/

as a spice used in foods). Curcumin as a supplement is proven to lower inflammation if enough is taken. [221]

Glutathione: The master antioxidant produced by your body. Glutathione can become depleted with Hashimoto's as with any chronic illness or detoxing of toxins/heavy metals.[222] Glutathione protects you from damage caused by Hashi's inflammation. It also helps with detoxifying. (My levels went quite low due to detoxing high heavy metals. I brought it back with shots, as it's a very important antioxidant.)

Inositol: Also called vitamin B8. It's stated that about 600 mg with 200 mg selenium can reduce antibodies in Hashi's patients and potentially reduce hypothyroidism. [223] [224]

Keto / Ketogenic: A very low-carb, high fat diet, where the body turns fat into ketones to use as your energy source.[225] Not everyone can handle how low the carb count is, but you can adjust for your needs.

LDN/Low Dose Naltrexone: This is a compounded medication. It's anti-inflammatory, a pain reliever, and has a great record for bringing down thyroid antibodies for most.[226] [227] Common starting dose is 0.5mg, increased by the same each week until reaching 4.5 mg. Some do well enough at 3 mg.[228] It can block the good effect of pain medications.

---

[221] https://examine.com/supplements/curcumin/
[222] https://drknews.com/glutathione-autoimmune-disease/
[223] https://www.ncbi.nlm.nih.gov/pmc/articles/PMC5331475/
[224] https://thyroidpharmacist.com/articles/myo-inositol-and-hashimotos/
[225] https://drjockers.com/ketogenic-diet-hypothyroid/
[226] http://stopthethyroidmadness.com/ldn
[227] https://www.ncbi.nlm.nih.gov/pmc/articles/PMC3962576/
[228] https://www.ldnresearchtrust.org/what-is-ldn

Lugol's Iodine: This is a liquid version of iodine with the combination of iodine and potassium iodide. There are 2% and 5% concentration of Lugols. With the 5%, one drop is said to equal 6.25 mg iodine. It can be stirred into a healthy drink of your choice. I personally do well and have for years on 12.5.

Natural Cleaners: These are cleaners devoid of chemicals like perchloroethylene / tetrachloroethylene (found in dry cleaning), phthalates (endocrine disruptors), quaternary ammonium (found in softener liquids or sheets), triclosan (found in anti-bacterial soaps, liquid or hard), etc. Natural cleaners may instead use vinegar, tea tree oil, baking soda, essential oils.

NAC: This stands for N-acetyl cysteine and is a supplement form of cysteine. NAC is a precursor for glutathione—the master antioxidant made by the body which can become depleted in Hashi's patients. It's wise to start low.

Natural Desiccated Thyroid: (NDT)   The oldest successful medication to treat hypothyroidism. Usually made from porcine if by prescription; bovine if over the counter. Contains the same five hormones as made by a healthy thyroid.[229]

NP Thyroid: This is a version of Natural Desiccated Thyroid made by Acella Pharmaceuticals, LLC[230]

Paleo / Paleo diet: Less strict than the Autoimmune Paleo. Based on foods that "cavemen" might have eaten, i.e. those from the Paleolithic era and the hunter/gatherer diet. High protein with meats, fish, fresh veggies, non-starch fruits, etc.[231]

[229] http://stopthethyroidmadness.com/natural-thyroid-101
[230] https://www.acellapharma.com/
[231] https://thepaleodiet.com/the-paleo-diet-premise/

Selenium: Soil-based mineral that has shown to help lower anti-TPO antibodies. Safe levels are stated to be at 200 - 400 mcg. Many find success at 200 mg. Supports the immune system, lowers inflammation. Also found in brazil nuts but with varying amounts depending on the soil where they were grown.

Transfer factors: These are small immune messenger molecules that are produced by all higher organisms. They are stated to be able to modulate an overreactive immune system[232]. Colostrum (what a mother releases from her breasts the first few weeks) is a known carrier of immune-modulating transfer factors. There are a variety of bovine and dried colostrum supplements.

Wobenzym: This is systemic enzyme formula with plant-derived enzymes bromelain and papain, stated to help lower inflammation.[233]

---

[232] https://www.ncbi.nlm.nih.gov/pubmed/23746171
[233] https://en.wikipedia.org/wiki/Wobenzym

NOTES

: # Chapter 17

The Journey to Remission: You Can Do It!

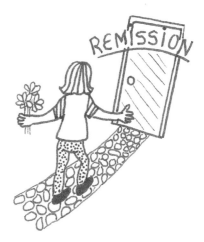

Compared to a few years ago, there are now very successful ways to reverse the progression of Hashimoto's. It's all evidenced by a growing body of informed Hashimoto's patients and all advocates who have contributed to the knowledge. **Being informed and proactive is key!**

Here is a summarized list of ways to deal with Hashi's based on years of patient reports and experiences, plus excellent info from research and other sources.

PART ONE
For Those in the Exploration Phase (no diagnosis yet,
but wondering or suspicious)

1. **Start early!** If you see any family history of autoimmune diseases, or if you already have other autoimmune issues yourself, regularly get the two main Hashimoto's antibodies tested. Don't join the slew of others who unknowingly went years before realizing they had it.

2. **Even if you don't have a noticeable family history of autoimmune disease,** or have no autoimmune problem yourself, get both antibodies tested anyway. Find out!

3. **Don't allow your doctor to order only ONE thyroid antibody test.** Make sure you test both anti-TPO and anti-Tg (thyroglobulin), since one can be high and the other isn't. You also want both in order to monitor your progress in getting either or both down. Some patients with both will see one go down, and the other still high. You need to know.

4. **Even if neither of the antibodies shows a problem, yet you notice thyroid swelling, talk to your doctor about an ultrasound, just in case.** There is a form of Hashi's that shows no antibodies called Seronegative Hashimoto's, also mentioned in Chapter 6.

5. **Have you noticed days where you're feeling hypo, then days you were feeling hyper, and back and forth?** That could be a sign of the attack in Hashimoto's disease. Get both thyroid antibodies for a baseline as to what is going on.

6. **Start early in noticing if certain foods give you trouble.** Pay attention to your reactions to certain foods. Gluten is a huge trigger,

but so can other foods that you react to. They can all make Hashi's and the antibodies worse. Study patient reports of reactions to foods in Chapter 13.

7. **Truly find ways to lower your stress** since it can be a trigger towards seeing Hashi's raise its autoimmune head. There are many ways, like gentle yoga, walking, easy jogging, doing what you love, hobbies, singing, avoiding toxic people the best you can at work or home, taking naps, deep breathing, a full night's sleep, and meditation…on and on. Find your way!

8. **Consider immune supportive supplements that you know you tolerate** to counter a viral or bacterial infection, as infections can be a trigger towards developing Hashimoto's disease or making it far worse. Examples are Vitamin C, colostrum, monolaurin, probiotics, whole food vitamins and more.

9. **Keep your Vitamin D levels optimal,** which also improves and modulates your immune function. Too many Hashi's patients find their level was low. More triggers are found in Chapter 4. If you feel bad on Vitamin D, time to check your parathyroid hormones and calcium level, the latter which should be no higher than midrange. *https://stopthethyroidmadness.com/parathyroid* Poor mineral levels are a second cause, as well.

10. **Treat any inflammation!** Inflammation from any cause is a trigger for developing Hashimoto's or making things worse. *https://stopthethyroidmadness.com/inflammation*i   Also see Chapter 8.

11. **Read what is below as well.**

PART TWO
For Those Who Already Have the Diagnosis or
Strongly Suspect Hashi's

FOODS YOU CONSUME

There are such a strong body of Hashimoto's patients with food issues that are making their Hashi's and antibodies worse that it's an important area to consider.

1. **If you haven't already, be committed to getting off all gluten,** as the vast majority react badly to it and see an increase of their antibodies. See patient reactions to gluten in Chapter 13.

2. **Watch out for gluten cross-contamination!** They can include gluten-free foods which have been exposed to gluten foods, or items in your kitchen like cutting boards, knives, pots and pans. Even be aware that store-bought corn and rice may have be prepared in facilities that have gluten products. Same with some oats.

3. **Be aware of the following foods. Though it's individual, these are the most problematic as reported by Hashimoto's patients:** eggs, sugar, dairy, soy, nightshades like tomatoes, potatoes, eggplant, bell peppers, corn, alcohol, nuts, beans…you name it. Having a bad reaction plus the inflammation it causes can make you worse with your overreactive immune system. See Chapter 13.

4. **On the other side of the food coin, focus on more nutrient rich foods in your diet** which promotes better health overall. They can include fresh vegetables, berries, healthy fats (olive oil, avocados, coconut oil), yogurt and more. In fact, eating like this can save you money by cutting down certain supplements.

5. **Learn about different ways to eat overall.** They are reported by many patients as having changed their lives. They are the GAPS diet, Autoimmune Paleo (AIP) diet, Paleo diet, and Low FODMAP diet. See the last pages in Chapter 13 for explanation of all of them.

GUT ISSUES

Problems in your stomach and intestines can be strong issues in making your symptoms worse.

6. **Read and study all the information about gut issues** in Chapters 9 and 10. It's detailed and important information.

7. **Have poor levels of digestive enzymes?** Or just want to improve the breakdown of your food? Time to consider digestive enzymes. Read HASHIMOTO'S GUT PROBLEM #1: Poor Levels of Digestive Enzymes in Chapter 9, page 93.

8. **Have low stomach acid?** This is important to treat as low levels cause problems in the breakdown and release of nutrients. It's all too common for stomach acid to go down when hypothyroid, treated with T4-only medications like Synthroid or Levothyroxine, or underdosed on natural desiccated thyroid or T3 due to a doctor's misinformed reliance on the TSH lab test. Read HASHIMOTO'S GUT PROBLEM #2 pages 95-97.

9. **The use of probiotics may be important.** We need a good bacterial community in our gut for good health and well-being. Read pages 123-126.

10. **Do you have a leaky gut?** Study the last section in Chapter 10 titled HASHIMOTO'S GUT PROBLEM #9: Leaky Gut and how to treat, page 127.

11. **What if you have parasites?** Parasites are not common, but they can enter your intestinal tract and are a trigger to make you worse. See the last Gut Health section, #8, pgs 110-112.

12. **Having an optimal release of bile is important.** If your gall-bladder isn't releasing enough bile, or you don't have a gallbladder, the ability to breakdown fat and toxins can be inhibited. Symptoms of a gallbladder issue can be poorly formed stools, smelly stools, diarrhea after eating, gas, etc. See your doctor if you have any reason to be suspicious.

INFLAMMATION

Hashimoto's equals inflammation. Though normal inflammation has an important purpose, the kind of chronic inflammation that Hashi's patients can get from the attack on the thyroid can promote more inflammation and become a very, serious issue.

13. **It can be important to avoid or seriously curtail inflammation-promoting foods.** Chronic inflammation is not something you want to continue feeding, as it triggers worsening problems. Those foods can include most grains, dairy, nightshades, sugar, eggs, gluten and corn for most, but there can be exceptions. Read HASHIMOTO'S GUT PROBLEM #3: Consuming Inflammation-Promoting Foods, pgs 98-99.

14. **While working on any causes of inflammation, consider using anti-inflammatory supplements** if you know you tolerate

them. Many are listed here: *http://stopthethyroidmadness.com/ inflammation*   But also see what I mention in #20 in this list.

TREATMENT OF ONE'S HYPOTHYROID STATE

Hashimoto's can be sneaky. And before you know it, you have a damaged thyroid causing hypothyroidism.

15. **Did you know that the wrong thyroid meds can make your gut problems worse?** Those wrong medications are T4-only like Synthroid, Levothyroxine, Eltroxin and Oroxine, etc. Why is that stated? It's about years and years of patient use and reported experiences. T4 is simply a storage hormone, and you miss getting all five thyroid hormones. Thus, being on just a storage hormone has caused numerous problems, one of which is lowered stomach acid. When stomach acid is low, nutrients aren't absorbed well and will fall. This is covered at HASHIMOTO'S GUT PROBLEM #5: The Wrong Thyroid Medications in Chapter 9.

16. **Using the right thyroid medication is needed to truly feel better and get out of one's hypothyroid state!** They include natural desiccated thyroid, synthetic T4/T3, or just T3. And remember they are about achieving optimal lab results, not just being "on them". This page explains: *http://stopthethyroidmadness.com/lab-values*

17. **To raise natural desiccated thyroid or T3 successfully and without problems**, it's important to have optimal levels of iron and cortisol. For women, optimal serum iron gets them close to 110 (or 23 in some Canadian or European ranges). For men, optimal always seems to put their serum iron in the mid-to-upper 130's (or close to the top of range in Canadian or European ranges

that end at 30). *Read http://stopthethyroidmadness.com/iron-and-cortisol*

ADRENALS and THYROID

Unfortunately, the stress of the autoimmune attack plus being in an untreated or poorly treated hypothyroid state can promote cortisol problems.

18. **Consider ordering a 24-hour cortisol saliva test** to find out if you have a cortisol problem[234] [235]   Here's an affiliated link: *https://tinyurl.com/saliva-cortisol*   Then compare your results to the following page, not just to what the facility says: *https://stopthethyroidmadness.com/lab-values*   See Chapter 11 for more info about adrenals.

19. **Treat a cortisol problem,** since too high or too low cortisol can make Hashimoto's worse. Chapter 11 has information based on patient experiences and wisdom. Treatments are explained in Chapters 5 and 6 of the updated revision Stop the Thyroid Madness book (with the byline of A Patient Revolution Against Decades of Inferior Thyroid Treatment). Please work with your doctor with all the information.

20. **If you know you do NOT have a cortisol problem** (you wake up feeling refreshed and it lasts all morning, you fall asleep fast at bedtime, you stay asleep all night), don't forget to be kind to your adrenals during any life stress. There are adaptogenic herbs that can help calm the adrenals during stress like

---

[234] http://stopthethyroidmadness.com/adrenal-info
[235] http://stopthethyroidmadness.com/saliva-cortisol

Ashwaghanda or adaptogen mixes.

EXPOSURE TO HEAVY METALS OR CHEMICALS

21. **If you are being chronically exposed to high levels of heavy metals, they can negatively affect your liver and gallbladde**r. Ask your water company for a breakdown of what's in your water, especially lead and other metals. Look into a water filter to be safe. Check your RBC zinc levels, as low zinc will cause copper to raise. Have a lot of silver dental fillings? This can cause high levels of mercury. E-cigarettes may contain too much cadmium.

22. **Household chemicals, pesticides and more toxins can be lurking in your life.**[236] Thus, some Hashi's patients are removing these kind of products and using organic, plant-based, hypo-allergenic, eco-friendly and non-toxic cleaning supplies or pesticides. Do an internet search for these.

INFECTIONS or ILLNESSES

23. **Create a better resistance to illnesses, because they can make Hashi's worse, report patients.** Eat healthier foods (those you tolerate), avoiding processed foods, treat any and all gut issues (Chapters 9 and 10), exercise weekly (even if it's walking), go to bed when you are tired...don't fight it, find a way to get your own needed amount of sleep hours, keep positive people in your life and keep a distance from toxic people to the degree that you can, avoid toxins.

ANTIBODIES

24. **Get those antibodies down!** Chapter 16 has many patient-reported ways to do so. Find what works for you! Page 199+.

---

[236] https://www.consciouslifestylemag.com/harmful-chemicals-and-toxins/

25. **Look into Low Dose Naltrexone (LDN)** if antibodies are very stubborn. It has proven to be very successful for the majority or patients. LDN is compounded. See *http://stopthethyroidmadness.com/ldn* plus more info at the end of Chapter 16.

NUTRIENT LEVELS

26. **How are your iron levels?**[237] No, this is not just about ferritin, which is simply storage iron. This is about all four iron labs, with serum iron being your most important focus when it comes to iron levels. We test serum iron, % saturation, TIBC, and ferritin. More info here: *http://stopthethyroidmadness. com/iron*

27. **Wbat about B12?**[238] This needs to be optimal to help you feel better. It's simply too common when Hashimoto's has caused thyroid damage to see B12 go down (just like iron). Optimal puts B12 in the upper quarter of the range. See *http://stopthethyroidmadness.com/b12*

28. **Keeping Vitamin D optimal is important for modulating and improving your immune function.** Optimal D may slow the progression of Hashi's, and decrease heart and artery problem risks. Vitamin K can direct calcium to your bones. Vitamin D3 is the supplement of choice. If you feel bad with adding vitamin D3, it can point to a parathyroid problem: *http://stopthethyroidmadness.com/parathyroid*

29. **For some patients, their judicious use of iodine supplementa- tion helped lower high antibodies.** Iodine use by Hashimoto's

---

[237] http://stopthethyroidmadness.com/iron
[238] http://stopthethyroidmadness.com/b12

patients can be about low and slow to counter the natural detox we encounter from the iodine, since that detox can raise antibodies in some. Selenium, magnesium, B2/B3 and salt supplementation is used to help counter the detox[239]. It's not about high amounts of iodine for most. If there is concern as to whether you need iodine, ask your doctor if you can tolerate an Iodine Loading Test. And as always, do you own research to decide if iodine use is for you!

30. **Want to test your nutrient levels, since with Hashi's, it's important to have good levels?** I love the Spectracell Micronutrient test[240]. It measures 31 vitamins, minerals, amino/fatty acids, antioxidants, and metabolites. Since putting Hashi's into remission is also about being as healthy as possible, having the right amount of nutrients is key. *https://www.spectracell.com/micronutrient-test-panel/*

STRESS

31. **Stress is your enemy with Hashimoto's**[241]. Though we can't always avoid it, we can moderate our lives to deal with stress better or find ways to remove or limit stressful people. Why is stress so bad? It can raise cortisol, which can cause an increase in reverse T3, the inactive hormone. The latter makes you more hypothyroid, and being more hypothyroid can stress the adrenals all over again. Then you risk the high cortisol plummeting to low cortisol. Stress can also negatively affect your immune system...the worst thing you want.

---

[239] https://stopthethyroidmadness.com/2013/12/29/companion-nutrients-the-key-to-iodine-protocol/
[240] https://www.spectracell.com/micronutrient-test-panel/
[241] https://www.ncbi.nlm.nih.gov/pubmed/15650357

LET'S TALK THYROID MEDICATIONS

• •

Important note: we need to have "optimal" levels of iron and cortisol, not just "in range", to avoid problems when raising any of the below. See *https://stopthethyroidmadness.com/iron-and-cortisol* to understand optimal levels.

In order of preference according to years of reported patient experiences and the wisdom gained from those experiences:

1. Natural Desiccated Thyroid (NDT)—a wise choice

This is a porcine-derived thyroid glandular by prescription which comes from an inspected mix of porcine glands, then dried, powdered, and pressed into tablets. NDT was first used around the 1890's, so it's been tried and true a long time. Pig is used because its tissue is compatible with humans.

NDT, like the human thyroid, contains five well-known thyroid hormones: T4, T3, T2, T1 and calcitonin. One grain of NDT, which is often 60 mg, is 38 mcg T4 and 9 mcg T3, with unmeasured amounts of T2, T1 and calcitonin. Some grains are 65 mg with just slightly different amounts of the measured T4 and T3. More in Chapter 2 of the updated revised Stop the Thyroid Madness book.

Popular US brands can include NP Thyroid by Acella Pharmaceuticals LLC or Armour by Allergan˙ and their affiliate Forest Laboratories, LLC.

Sometimes ownership changes. Sometimes new versions come out. There are other brands like WP Thyroid by RLC labs and more. Countries like Australia and New Zealand use compounded NDT.

There are some over-the-counter versions such as Thyroid-S, Thiroyd, Thyrogold, Thyrovanz, and various ones sold on the internet or in vitamin or health food stores. Those are mostly bovine. The FDA hates them: patients love them.

A safe amount of NDT as a starting dose is one grain for most, though there may be variations made by one's doctor. Raises of 30 mg. occur every two weeks or so, slowing down in the 2-3 grain area to redo lab work, say patients. Optimal amounts of NDT seem to put the free T3 towards the top part of the range, and the free T4 around midrange. Both, say patient reports. TSH will naturally fall below range.

NDT is often taken twice a day, such as morning and early afternoon. Many patients place it under their tongue; others chew or swallow.

If there are problems when raising NDT like fast heartrate, anxiety, etc., it points to:

a) staying on too low a dose (which increases adrenaline over time and can cause cortisol problems), or

b) having non-optimal amounts of iron and/or cortisol. Four iron labs are needed (serum iron, % saturation, TIBC and ferritin). Cortisol testing is via saliva, not blood. Optimal results are important, not just in range: *http://stopthethyroidmadness.com/lab-values*

More info about saliva testing is here: http://stopthethyroidmadness. com/saliva-cortisol

More excellent info on Natural Desiccated Thyroid in Chapter 2 of the updated revised STTM book: *http://laughinggrapepublishing.com*

2. Synthetic T4 with Synthetic T3—another good choice

For those who have a problem with pork, or an uninformed doctor who refuses to prescribe NDT, using both synthetic T4 with synthetic T3 has been a good choice. See info below concerning brand names for T4 and T3.

With raises of both, the eventual goal of using the two synthetics is the same as with NDT: the free T3 towards the top part of the range, and the free T4 around midrange. Both, say years of patient observations. There may be slight variations. Again, we have to have "optimal" amounts of iron and cortisol to avoid problems when raising.

T4 can be taken once a day, but it's better to take T3 at two other times a day due to its short half-life.

If there are problems with raising either, especially T3, such as high heartrate, palpitations, or anxiety, read the information in #1 about those problems and why they can occur.

3. Synthetic T3-only (triiodothyronine)—3rd choice

T3 is the active thyroid hormone which takes away hypothyroid symptoms when one is optimal on T3-only meds. T3 is usually dosed up to 3 times a day due to its short half-life. Examples of brand names include Cytomel, Liothyronine Sodium (generic— one example is Sigma Pharm among many others), Tiromel, Tertroxin, Triostat, Cynomel and more.,

Two main reasons a Hashimoto's patient might only be on T3:

a) Having a genetic variation that causes problems with T4 converting to T3. One example is an active mutation in the DIO1 gene (Iodothyronine Deiodinase 1) Genetic testing can help.

b) If one's reverse T3 (RT3) is going up from the bottom 2-3 numbers in any range. RT3 is the inactive hormone made from T4, and if it goes up, one's chronic autoimmune inflammation can be one cause, as can high cortisol from stress. Another cause is having low levels of iron due to being undiagnosed hypothyroid, poorly treated hypothyroidism from T4, or held to the TSH on any thyroid med. RT3 is covered here: *http://stopthethyroidmadness.com/reverse-t3*

The free T3 lab result on T3-only, when optimal and having the right amount of cortisol, ends up at the top of range, report patients. Some patients report they are slightly over range and doing well. It's individual.

Patients have learned that if cortisol is low, the free T3 can go high with continuing hypo symptoms, called pooling. Cortisol is needed to get T3 to your cells. See *http://stopthethyroidmadness. com/pooling* It's a good reason to do the saliva cortisol test, then compare the results to the Lab Values page on the Stop the Thyroid Madness website.

4. Synthetic T4-only (thyroxine)—not the best choice, say patients

This medication--actually the least effective if used by itself, say many patients over the years--was first produced in the 1920's, but hit the promotional market more strongly around 1960. The first commercial name was Synthroid by Knoll Pharmaceuticals of Germany.

Over the years, doctors fell for the marketing of only T4, putting the vast majority of thyroid or Hashimoto's patients on it. But it failed millions sooner or later, forcing the body to live for conversion alone to T3, which a healthy thyroid would never do to you. Thus, it has resulted in millions having symptoms of continued hypothyroidism, sooner or later.

On the next page are common lingering symptoms as expressed by patients from being on T4-only...sooner or later. You will note they are the same as hypothyroid symptoms.

Less stamina than others	Easy weight gain
Less energy than others	Inability to lose
Deep exhaustion	Aching bones/muscles
Long recovery period after activity	Osteoporosis
Bad reaction to exercise	Bumps on legs
Frequent napping	Painful soles of feet
Inability to hold children for long	Poor skin quality
Arms feeling heavy after activity	Hives
Chronic low-grade depression	Swelling
Chronic severe depression	Heart palps
The need for anti-depressants	Exhaustion in every dimension– physical, mental, spiritual, emotional
Suicidal thoughts	Slowing to a snail's pace
Often feeling cold	Illegible handwriting
Cold hands or feet	Internal itching of ears
High cholesterol	Weak fingernails
Being on Statins	Anxiety
Colitis	Ringing in ears
Days without a BM	Inability to eat in the mornings
Constipation	Joint pain
Hard little round stools	Carpal tunnel symptoms
Painful bladder	No appetite
Loss of outer eyebrows	Heart Fluid retention
Dry hair	Swollen legs that prevented walking
Dry skin	Blood Pressure problems
Cracked heels	Rising cholesterol levels
Ridged fingernails	Inner Ear problems
Hair loss	Low body temperature
White new hair growth	Tightness in throat; sore throat
Hair breaks faster than it grows	Swollen lymph glands
Nodding off	Overreaction to cold medications
Requires naps in the afternoon	Allergies worsening
Sleep Apnea	
Air Hunger	

Inability to concentrate	Sleepiness at work
Forgetfulness	A cold rear end
Foggy thinking	Irritable bowel syndrome
Relationship problems	Dysphagia Nerve Damage, aka
NO sex drive	(inability to swallow food)
Moody	Pneumonia
Crabby	Easy sicknesses
PMS	Being sick longer
Heavy period	Slow to recover from illness
Failure to ovulate and/or	High adrenaline release
constant bleeding	Overactive Autonomic Nervous
Problems getting pregnant	System (Dysautonomia)
Worsening PTSD (post-traumatic	Adrenal stress
stress disorder)	Adrenal fatigue (low cortisol)
Inability to work full time	High cortisol

Staying hypothyroid, which T4-only has caused with millions sooner or later, can cause stress which makes Hashimoto's disease worse, besides stress on one's adrenals, plus the lowering of nutrients due to low stomach acid.

5. Compounded Thyroid Medications

This is a method of having your thyroid meds made via specialized pharmacies. Patients can choose their own fillers like olive oil or vitamin C, to name a few. Often, compounded thyroid medications are slow release, which hasn't always worked well, say some patients. You can request immediate release in order to multi-dose. Compounded can be the most expensive way to have thyroid medications, but some patients appreciate choosing their own fillers.

TSH, THE POINTLESS LAB TEST

· ·

Because of the autoimmune attack on the thyroid, many Hashimoto's patients will find themselves with hypothyroidism. Yet, if a doctor simply goes by the TSH lab test, your hypothyroidism can remain undiagnosed for years!

The TSH lab test was created around 1973. It's based on the real Thyroid Stimulating Hormone, a messenger hormone released by your pituitary gland. It's part of a messaging feedback loop between the hypothalamus in your brain, to the pituitary in your brain, to your thyroid...telling your thyroid to produce and release thyroid hormones. And back again.

But guess what patients have noticed repeatedly?

It can take years before the TSH lab test rises high enough to reveal one's hypothyroid state, all while your hypothyroidism is making you worse! So due to your doctor's uninformed reliance on this lousy test, you could remain undiagnosed and untreated. That means more stress on your Hashimoto's, as well as increased problems with your gut health from low stomach acid.

Additionally, if the TSH is used to ascertain the "right" amount of either natural desiccated thyroid, T4/T3, or T3 alone, you can stay hypothyroid!

It is very normal for the TSH lab test result to go below range as you are raising to find your optimal amount of these thyroid medications, yet doctors think you are overdosed. So, they lower the amount you are on to raise the TSH, and you become more hypothyroid---more stress to the autoimmune Hashimoto's, and especially gut health!

Why is the TSH lab test so counter to what is going on?

Because for diagnosis, different organs manage thyroid hormones differently, i.e. though one organ will get enough, another won't.

Additionally, while on NDT, T4/T3 or T3, having a TSH below range is simply indicative that our thyroid medications are taking over the job of the actual TSH, so it falls low in the man-made range. And that does NOT mean autoimmune Graves' disease—a hyperthyroid state which also pushes the TSH quite low.

Why does my doctor proclaim I will get heart problems or bone loss with my low TSH while on these medications?

Doctors confuse the low TSH while on NDT, T4/T3 or T3 to the low TSH with autoimmune Graves' disease. And uncontrolled Graves' can cause heart problems or bone loss. But the low TSH while on the latter medications is totally different. And to the contrary, when we get optimal, patients report improved heart and bone health.

What are better tests for diagnosis or the use of NDT, T4/T3 or T3?

The free T3 and free T4 are superior. Less than midrange, that's hypothyroidism. For optimal treatment, we seek a free T3 towards the top part of the range, and a free T4 midrange. Both. But we have to have optimal iron and cortisol to get there without problems. We also look at the RT3 (reverse T3)—it should be at the bottom 2-3 numbers in any range. On T3-only, patients only look at the free T3.

Is there anything good about the TSH lab test?

Yes! If not on thyroid medications, *and both the TSH and free T3 are low,* that can point to hypopituitary, also called pituitary insufficiency. This is a less common condition where your pituitary gland fails to release certain messenger hormones like **TSH**. It can also affect other messenger hormones like **ACTH** (stimulates your adrenals to produce cortisol and affects your blood pressure), **FSH** and **LH** (influences the testes and ovaries in the production of testosterone and estrogen), **GH** growth hormone (promotes normal growth of your bones and tissue), **ADH** antidiuretic hormone (helps controls the water loss by your kidneys), and **Prolactin** hormone (stimulates milk production and female breast growth).

Other than finding hypopituitary, the use of the TSH for diagnosis or finding the right amount of NDT, T4/T3 or T3 is the fool's errand

For the TSH, see *http://stopthethyroidmadness.com/tsh-why-its-useless*

15 Ways
to Handle Stress

● ●

Some experts state that stress alone is a strong predictor for the onset of Hashimoto's. And patients know from experience that stress can definitely make active Hashimoto's worse, causing flares. Look at it this way: stress causes your body to produce more adrenaline and cortisol. Cortisol will rise higher and higher, causing all sorts of problems including rising reverse T3, the inactive hormone. Then the high cortisol can fall to low cortisol. Low cortisol is full of stressful problems!

So, let's talk about several ways to manage your life stresses.

1. Go to sleep when your body tells you to go to sleep, and sleep enough hours

There is a reason your body makes you feel sleepy in the evening—it wants you to sleep! Sleep has important functions. It promotes a better immune function for one, which is crucial for Hashimoto's patients. It helps your brain's cognitive abilities and memory. It improves your skeletal, nervous and muscular systems. Sleep restores you! That's all why it's important to listen to your body and go to bed, besides get in the hours of sleep that experience has told you that you need.

2.   Have insomnia?

Insomnia is usually caused by high bedtime cortisol. And there are excellent supplements to consider to knock that high cortisol down, say patients, which are holy basil (if you tolerate it), Phosphatidyl Serine, or even zinc. Other herbs which might help include chamomile, valerian root, lavender and magnesium—please research them. Since low cortisol can also cause insomnia in a few, that's why doing a 24-hour adrenal saliva test can help discern as to what is going on.

3.   Talk to someone

As simple as it sounds, talking to someone you trust can be a great stress-reliever. Think of a friend or family member you can do that with. There are even online therapy websites for a fee.

4.   Set aside time to do things you love

This is actually very important to do those activities that bring you joy, whether art, singing, watching a funny movie, reading a good book, walking, taking a drive to see the scenery, listening to music you love, you name it.

5.   **Decide what activities you can delegate to others**

Yes, it is actually possible that there are some daily tasks you do that someone else can do instead. Think on it. List your tasks, then decide if someone else might do some of them. Learn to say no where you can say no.

6.   **Meditation**

There are guided meditations on YouTube that can help you relax and refocus.

7.   **See if there are yoga or tai-chi classes near you.**

Either will promote needed relaxation, besides potential social contact.

8.   **Breathe...**

Taking deep breaths, hold, release...and again. This can be done anywhere and you'll be amazed how that can help relax you.

9.   **If you are able to walk, go walk.**

Walking can be a great stress reliever. Take your headset and listen to your favorite relaxing or uplifting music. If a street is too busy, use your driveway, property, hallways, or a safe place near where you live.

10.   **Make lunchtime at work a positive experience.**

Take foods you love. Eat outside. Sit by pleasant people. Leave your workspace for lunch.

11.   **Like to play board or card games? Play them with loved ones or friends.**

Playing a fun game is relaxing.

12. Gardening

For some, being in nature and planting provides great stress relief.

13. Stop the coffee drinking after lunch or afternoon

Caffeine can keep you awake plus push adrenaline up. Some even simply switch to decaffeinated coffee or tea even in the mornings. Explore instant hot chicory drink with cream and sweetener.

14. Play music and sing

Not only can the right kind of music relax you, singing has known benefits in lowering and releasing stress.

15. Get away with a mini-trip

Taking a mini-vacation also takes us away from stress. It can be relaxing, fun and distracting if done well.

MTHFR /
METHYLATION 101

．．．．．．．．．．．．．．．．．．．．．．．．．．．．．．．．

What the heck does methylation mean? Why is it important to
know for Hashimoto's patients?

Methylation is an "interior chemical process" that happens in your
cells and tissues. It means a particular molecule is added to another
substance so that the latter substance can function correctly. Having
your body function correctly is important when you already deal
with autoimmune diseases!

This methylation process helps all the following:
- Optimal functioning of nervous system
- Regulates immune system function
- Better cardiovascular health
- Detoxification of heavy metals
- Better energy
- Positively influences transmitters that affect your mood
- Improves your cognitive abilities
- Helps give you enough phosphatidylcholine, a composition of
  bile
- Helps your DNA/genetics work better

Thus, if your methylation process is not working right, you could have:

- Depression (also caused by over-methylation)
- Anxiety (also caused by over-methylation)
- Additional inflammation
- Rising heavy metals
- Faster aging
- Fatigue
- Brain problems
- Histamine rise causing allergies
- Infertility
- High B12 (not being broken down for use)
- High selenium
- Heart problems
- Stroke risk
- Obsessive-compulsive tendencies
- Sleep problems
- Digestive problems
- A variety of illnesses.

You can see that many of the latter can instigate Hashimoto's or make it worse!

What to test

1. **MTHFR Genes C677T and A1298C, also just called 677 and 1298** This is done via genetic testing such as 23andme.com, and the data received is uploaded to a site like livewello.com. Or you can request a blood test from your doctor. Just because you do have a mutation doesn't mean you have an active methylation problem. That's why it's important to look at your symptoms to

discern what is going on. If these genes have variants/mutations, and especially the 677, you won't convert folic acid to folate, the active form. It can cause high homocysteine, increasing the risk of heart disease or strokes. Homocysteine will not do a good job converting to glutathione, your master antioxidant and detoxifier, or convert to the important amino acid Methionine. Inflammation can go up—the worst thing you want to see with autoimmune Hashimoto's disease.

2. **Genes which can negatively affect methylation include like CBS, COMT, SUOX, MTRR and MTR, MOA-A and_MOA-B, AHCY, VDR, GPX.** This are also done via genetic testing such as 23andme.com, and the data received is uploaded to a site like livewello.com. Or ask your doctor.

3. **Key nutrients** Folate and B12 are strongly needed nutrients to support one's methylation process, but so are B2, B3, B6, zinc, choline, glutathione, magnesium, foods with sulphur, methionine, SAMe, and more.

Read more:
1. I have written about all the above more extensively: http://stopthethyroidmadness.com/mthfr
2. http://www.jillcarnahan.com/ has great info about methylation
3. The Kresser Institute has good info here: https://kresserinstitute.com/treating-methylation-supplementing/
4. https://suzycohen.com/articles/methylation-problems/

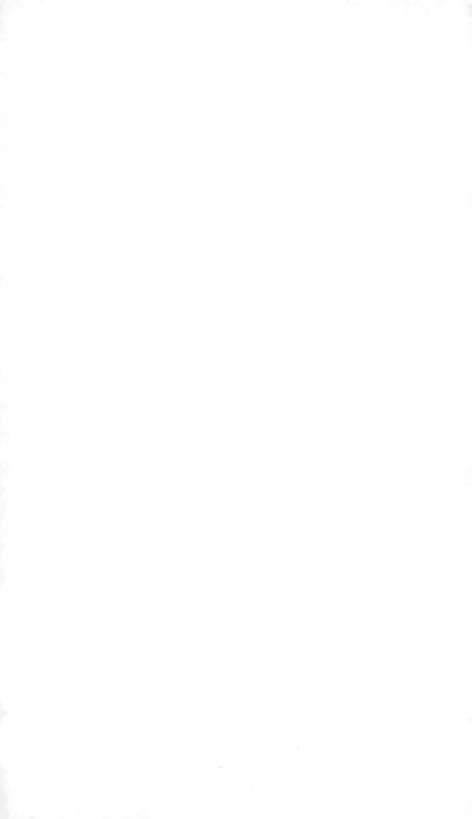

HOW PROBLEMATIC GUMS AND TEETH CAN HARM YOU WITH HASHIMOTO'S

• •

In 2017, I started having digestive problems. And I had no idea why, as I had never had problems like those before. I had to take betaine (hydrochloric acid) and digestive enzymes just to get by...barely.

It was a full year later that I found out why: *the root canal I had done about five years previous had an infection underneath it and I never knew it!* Thus, I was dropping infection down into my gut every time I swallowed. Imagine how this could affect YOU with autoimmunity tendencies like Hashimoto's!

As I thought back about getting that root canal, I wasn't impressed with the dentist back then. He seemed inexperienced. I also had a cap put on that tooth which felt awkward, and I had to go back to get him to fix it. I shudder to think about the fact that I could have had bacteria under that cap and in the root canal all that time! I can't prove it, but it seems logical, as I take good care of my teeth with frequent brushing.

What if YOU as a Hashi's patient have a problem like I had? That can only make things worse for you!

My experience is why I strongly recommend exploring going to biologic dentist. Biologic dentists may have a better understanding of how the health of your teeth and gums can impact your gut. They might also still do root canals, but they know how to do them safer.

In my situation, my biologic dentist removed the root canal, and he sprayed an anti-bacterial liquid in the cavity. I also remember the use of ozonated water somewhere in the procedure.

At another visit, he also removed a few of my amalgam fillings. That involved the use of a rubber covering (called a dam) placed in my mouth to prevent any flakes of the mercury amalgam from being swallowed. There was also a suction tube placed in my mouth during the procedure to keep vapors at bay.

If you have silver amalgams, there's mercury in there, too. And a buildup of internal mercury has the potential to activate Hashi's, say some experts, or make your active Hashi's worse. After removing a cavity, biologic dentists can fill a tooth in a healthier way, if you choose that direction. Do your research and decide what's right for you.

The bottom line is also to TAKE CARE of your teeth and gums as a Hashi's patient. There are excellent non-fluoridated and natural toothpastes, plus good electric or manual toothbrushes, and ways to remove food between the teeth with a Waterpik type device.

HASHIMOTO'S DOCTOR WISDOM

· ·

Q: What do you call a doctor who knows practically nothing about your Hashimoto's disease?

A: A doctor you don't want.

■

Q: What do you call a doctor who refuses to let you teach him/her what you know is good information for you?

A: A doctor you don't want.

■

Q: What do you call a doctor who only goes by the TSH lab test?

A: A doctor you don't want.

Q: What do you call a doctor who wants to only put you on T4 medications?

A: A doctor you don't want.

■

Q: What do you call a doctor who tells you not to listen to the internet or good books like this?

A: A doctor you don't want.

■

Q: What do you call a doctor who LISTENS to your wisdom and lets you be a PARTNER in your relationship with him or her?

A: A doctor you want to keep!!!

Index

B

C

P

CPSIA information can be obtained
at www.ICGtesting.com
Printed in the USA
FSHW021655100519

9 780985 615444